This book is dedicated to each of you for inspiring me. It is because of you sharing your concerns and your bravery to step up and be the voice for those who have been silenced that I am touched, inspired and driven to write this book sharing some of my most private secret recipes handed down for generations.

To your good health, live Strong

Find Your Inspiration

Finding Your Balance Of Health And Fitness

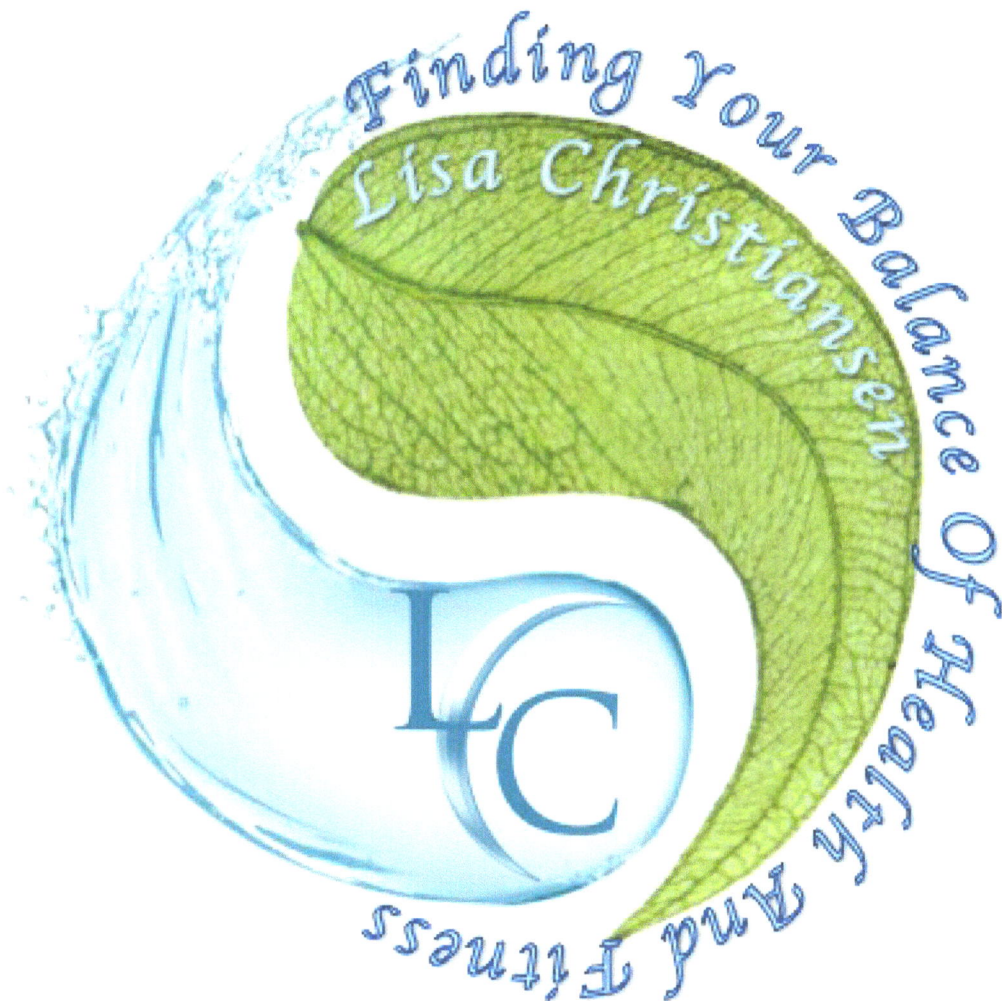

What is the difference between health and fitness?

The terms '**health**' and '**fitness**' are often used interchangeably these days, but there are important differences between them, even though they do interact. Let me explain.

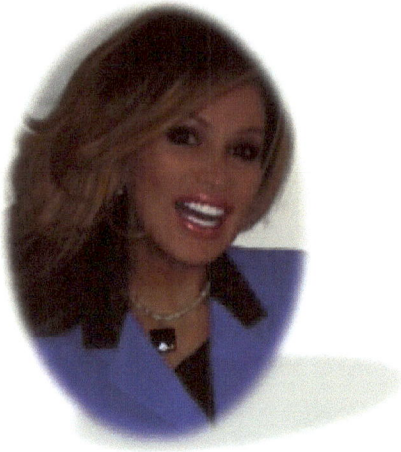

'Health' is a general term describing the overall status of a person. Being 'in good health' implies being free from illness or disease, and not suffering from any impairment or pain. It's rather vague, but being healthy does not necessarily mean that you are fit. And many things – food, environment, disease etc., and can affect health.

'Fitness' on the other hand, is more a measure of the amount of physical capability than a measure of well being. Fitness is almost entirely a result of action. Certainly food and drink can influence fitness. But the main way of increasing fitness is through exercise. And increasing your fitness has been shown to boost health is so many different ways -reduction in risk of cardiovascular disease, reduction in the risk of contracting many cancers, and boosting the immune system being just three of them.

It may seem like a question of semantics, but it IS important to know the difference between health and fitness. Being healthy is seen by most people as something that they can't influence.

- **You're either lucky to have good health, or you' re not, right?**

But fitness is something that is completely within the control of every person. Everyone (even Olympic athletes!) can improve his or her fitness by doing more of the correct sort of exercise. Vigorous cardiovascular exercise increases cardiovascular fitness, so that the more you do, the more you are able to do. Obviously you don't want to go overboard – that's a good way of getting injured. Just a steady progression of doing a little bit more each time you exercise.

And the best thing about it is that it is completely in your control.

- **You can't just be lucky and increase your fitness. You can only boost fitness by working at it.**

So you have a choice – either you want to improve your fitness (and as a additional benefit, your health) or you don't. If you do, you just need to do some work. If you don't, you can't blame any one or thing – you have just decided not to improve your health and fitness. Make no mistake – is really is a choice, but it's up to you which way to jump!

ᏣᎳᎩ ᎤᏪᏌ ᏗᏍᏋ

Heart Of The Cherokee

The most Important Recipe I Can Give You That I Created By Accident And God's Grace. Mix these ingredients in a blender. (Patent Pending #62112947)

This is what I call Drano for the arteries because it reduces cholesterol, keeps arteries pliable, cleans the plaque and reduces its ability to build up. It is a fat emulsifier eliminating fat through your waste, keeps your weight in balance. It will keep your skin smooth and it will give you energy. This has a fruit flavor with a hint of sweet nut.

½ cup Orange Juice

½ Cup Aloe Vera Juice

2 Tbs. Flax Seed Oil with Lignin

1 Tbs. Grapefruit Pectin

2 Tbs. Lecithin

1 Tbs. Royal Bee Jelly

1 Tbs. Bee Pollen

1 Tbs. Trail Of Tears Beans

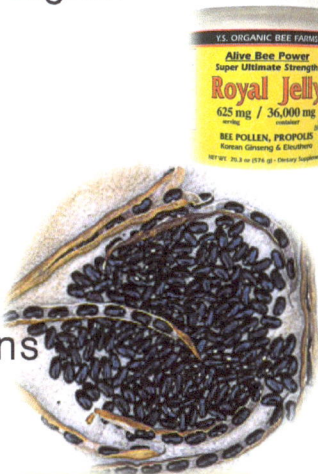

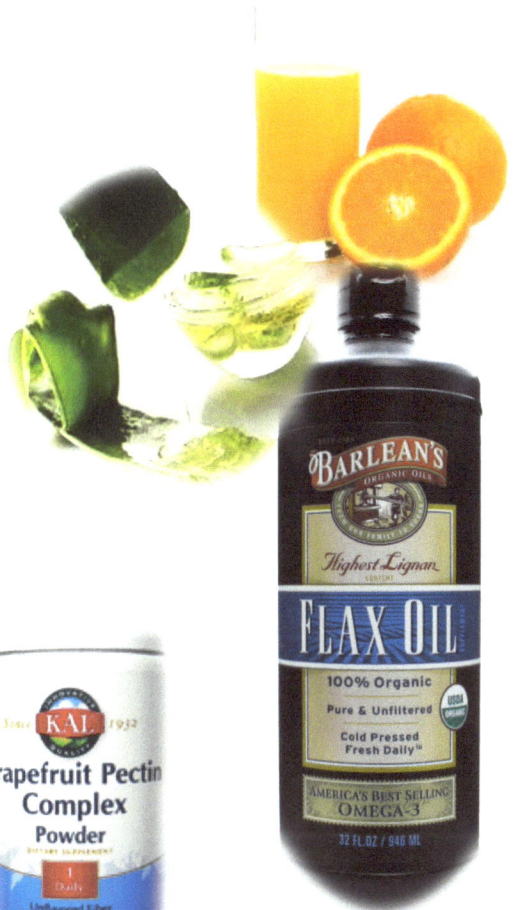

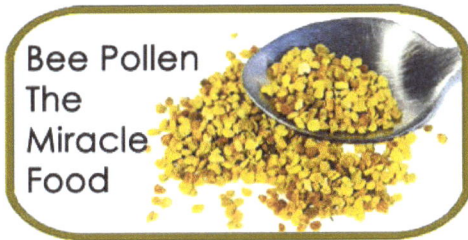

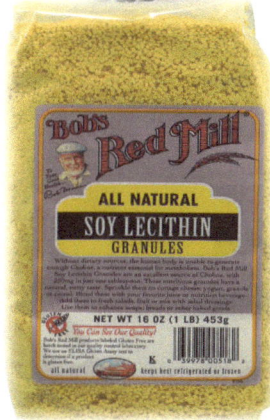

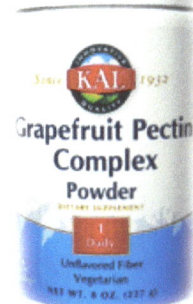

Winning Your Waist

Taking control is not about a diet it is a lifestyle change.

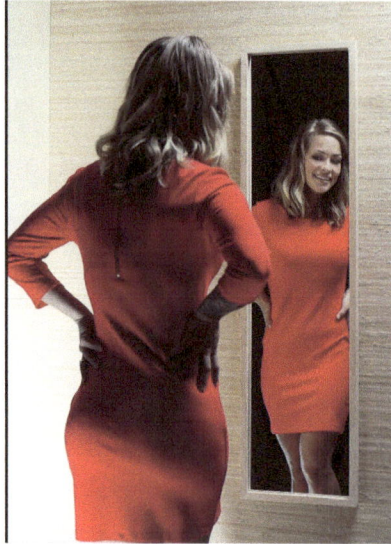

Supplement	Suggested Dosage
Very Important	
Aerobic Bulk Cleanse(ABC) from Aerobic Life Industries or psyllium husks	As directed on label. Always take supplemental fiber separately from other supplements and Medications. 1 tbsp. ½ hour before meals with a Large glass of liquid. Drink Quickly.
Chromium picolinate	200-600 mg. Daily
Essential fatty acids (flaxseed oil, primrose oil And salmon oil are good sources)	As directed on label
Kelp	1000-1500 mg. Daily
Lecithin granules or capsules	1 tbsp 3 times daily, before meals-1,200 mg 3 times daily, before meals
Spirulina or Spiru-tein from Nature's Plus	As directed on label 3 times daily- between meals
Vitamin C with bioflavonoids	3,000-6,000 mg. Daily

Helpful

Calcium	1,500 mg daily
Choline and Inositol	As directed on label
Coenzyme Q10	As directed on label
Dehydroeplandrosterone (DHEA)	As directed on label
Gamma-aminobulyric acid (GABA)	As directed on label
L-Arginine and L-ornithine plus L-lysine	500 mg each or as directed on label, before bed. Take on empty stomach with water or juice. Do Not take with milk. Take with 50 mg vitamin B6 And 100 mg vitamin C for better absorption.
L-Camitine	500 mg daily
L-Glutamine	As directed on label
L-Methionine	As directed on label
L-Phenylalanine	As directed on label, on an empty stomach
L-Tyrosine	As directed on label, take at bedtime
Maitake	As directed on label
Multivitamin and mineral complex with Potassium	As directed on label 99mg daily
Vitamin B complex plus extra Vitamin B2 (riboflavin) and Vitamin B3 (niacin)	50 mg 3 times daily 50 mg 3 times daily 50 mg 3 times daily-do not exceed this amt.
Vitamin B6 (pyridoxine) Vitamin B12	50 mg 3 times daily 50 mg 3 times daily
Zinc	80 mg daily. Do not exceed a total of 100mg Daily from all supplements

Herbs

Alfalfa, corn silk, dandelion, gravel root, horsetail, hydrangea, hyssop, juniper berries, oat straw, parsley, seawrack, thyme, uva ursi, white ash, and yarrow can be used in tea form for their diuretic properties.

Aloe vera juice improves digestion and cleanses the digestive tract.

Astragalus increases energy and improves nutrient absorption. (Don't take in presence of a fever).

Butcher's broom, cardamom, cayenne, cinnamon, Garcinia cambogia, ginger, green tea, and mustard seed are thermogenic herbs that improve digestion and aid in the metabolism of fat.(Don't use cinnamon in large quantities during pregnancy).

Bladder wrack, borage seed, hawthorn berry, licorice root, and sarsaparilla stimulate the adrenal glands and improve thyroid function.(If high blood pressure, avoid licorice. If overused it elevates blood pressure, do not use on a daily basis for more than seven days in a row.)

Ephedra, guarana, and kola nut are appetite suppressants(do not use ephedra if you suffer from anxiety, glaucoma, heart disease, high blood pressure, or insomnia, or if you are taking a monoamine oxidase (MAO) inhibitor drug for depression.

Fennel removes mucus and fat from the intestinal tract, and is a natural appetite suppressant.

Fenugreek is useful for dissolving fat within the liver.

Siberian ginseng aids in moving fluids and nutrients throughout the body, and reduces the stress of adjusting to new eating habits.(don't use if you have hypoglycemia, high blood pressure, or a heart disorder.)

Recommendations

Do not worry so much about the number of calories you consume as about eating the proper foods. Rotate your foods and be sure to eat a variety of foods. Eat meals that consist of a balance of proteins, complex carbohydrates, and some fat. By eating balanced meals you get more steady blood sugar levels and the ability to burn stored body fat for long-term weight loss.
Eat more complex carbohydrates that also offer protein, such as tofu, lentils, plain baked potatoes(no toppings, except for vegetables), sesame seeds, beans, brown rice, whole grains, skinless turkey or chicken breast and whitefish(no shellfish). Poultry and fish should be broiled or baked, never fried.
Eat fresh fruits and an abundance of raw vegetables. Try for 1 meal per day that consists only of vegetables and fruits. Use low-calorie vegetables such as broccoli, cabbage, carrots, cauliflower, celery, cucumbers, green beans, lettuce, onions, radishes, spinach and turnips. Good fruits are apples, cantaloupe, grapefruit, strawberries, and watermelon. Use less frequently bananas, cherries, corn, figs,

grapes, green peas, hominy,pears pineapple, sweet potatoes, white rice and yams. Eat foods raw, if possible. If heated, they should be baked, broiled, steamed or boiled. Avoid fried and greasy foods.

Drink 6-8 glasses of liquids daily. Herbal teas and steam-distilled water with trace minerals added are good. Herbal teas mixed with unsweetened fruit juice are good, use these between meals when a desire for sweets hits you. Drink sparkling water mixed with fruit juice in place of sodas.

Watch your fat intake, some is necessary, but make it the right kind. Avocados, olives, raw nuts and seeds, wheat germ are good. Do these in moderation (no more than twice a week. Eliminate saturated fats totally. Never consume animal fat, found in butter, cream, gravies, ice cream, mayo, meat, rich dressings, and whole milk. Don't eat fried food.

Consume in moderation- apples, brown rice, buckwheat, chestnuts, corn, grapes, oatmeal, white potatoes, and yellow vegetables. These contain small amounts of essential fatty acids

Good choices of snacks- celery and carrot sticks, low-fat cottage cheese topped with fresh applesauce and walnuts, unsweetened gelatin made with fruit juice in place of sugar and water, natural sugar-free whole-grain muffins, unsalted popcorn, watermelon, fresh fruit or frozen fruit popsicles, unsweetened low-fat yogurt topped with granola or nuts and fresh fruit.

Do not eat any white flour products, salt, white rice, or processed foods. Avoid fast food and junk food.

Do not consume sweets such as soda, pastries, pies, cakes, doughnuts, or candy. For a quick energy boost, try taking a Spirulina tablet Use wheatgrass to calm the appetite. Don't take alcohol in any form, including beer and wine. Use extra fiber daily. Guar gum and psyllium husks are good sources. Take fiber with large glass of liquid ½ hr. before meals. Be active, take a walk every day before breakfast or dinner. Use stairs instead of the elevator. Walk or ride a bike as opposed to driving, whenever possible. Get regular aerobic exercise, such as walking, running, bicycling, or swimming and do exercises for strength, such as yoga or stretching exercises. Be sure to drink water during exercise to prevent dehydration and cramps. If you have been sedentary for some time, try exercising in water.

Change your eating habits- Always eat breakfast. Eat small meals every 3-4 hrs., don't skip meals. Make your main meal lunch, not dinner. Some people don't consume food after 3:00 p.m. Put less food on your plate, chew slowly, stop eating as soon as you are no longer hungry. If you get the urge to eat, put on a tight belt, this will make you uncomfortable and remind you that you want to lose weight.
Learn to ride out your food cravings. They peak and subside like ocean waves. Tell yourself that you can satisfy the craving if you really want to. Then wait 10 minutes. Try to do something to distract yourself. If you decide to eat whatever, then decide how much is reasonable and enjoy it, take one bite and savor the taste, eat slowly. Find out what causes your cravings. If you like to eat, while watching TV, try reading, drinking a big glass of water or taking a walk. Do not grocery shop on an empty stomach, you will be tempted to buy forbidden foods Avoid crash dieting. To maintain weight loss, calculate how many calories you need daily by multiplying your weight by 10, then add 30 % (this # you can consume daily, without gaining back.

Considerations

The basic math of weight loss is that each pound of body fat is worth 3,500 calories. To lose 1 pound a week (a good, safe reasonable goal) you must tip the calorie consumption in your favor by 500 calories each day. To maintain weight loss, you must adopt a healthier, more active lifestyle. This includes a natural, healthy diet and regular exercise. Quick weight loss tends to come back rapidly. A study shows that using artificial sweeteners tend to cause weight gain, not lost. Calories derived from fat are more easily converted into flab than calories from other sources. The need to eat something sweet after a meal is an acquired habit and can be broken. Eating a low-fat diet that is high in complex carbohydrates does not mean eating tasteless, bland foods. The goal is to reduce the total fat, saturated fat, and cholesterol in the diet and to increase the amount of complex carbohydrates. Potatoes, pasta, breads, corn, rice and other complex-carbohydrates rich foods are not the cause of obesity, they are the cure.

Hydroxycitric acid (HCA) has proven very effective for weight management. It suppresses hunger and also helps to prevent the body from turning carbohydrate calories into fat. It is available in supplement form. Gamma-linoleic acid (GLA) helps to control the metabolism of fats. Taking at least 250IU of GLA a day helps to control the appetite. Diet Esteem Plus from Esteem is a diet product that contains many of the nutrients recommended plus the herbal extract HCA. Trace mineral boron may speed the burning of calories. Raisins and onions are good boron sources.

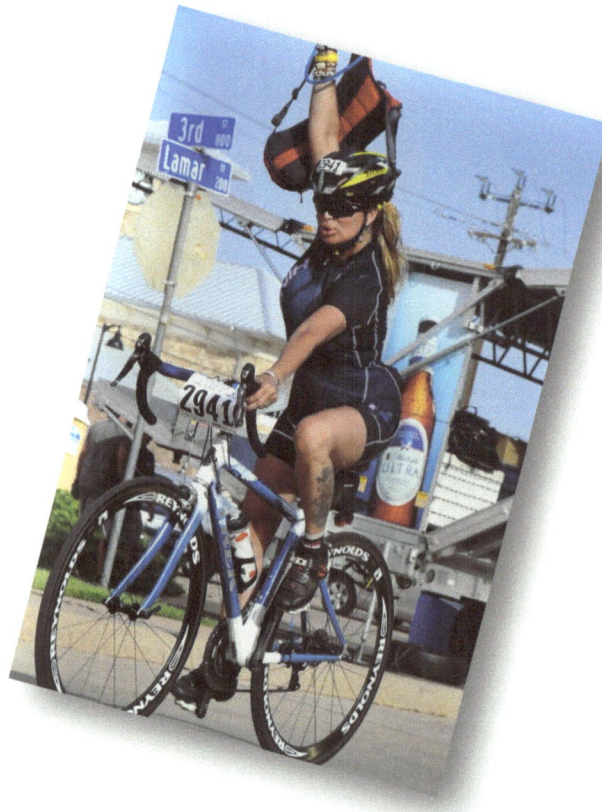

Cilantro is a phenomenal herb that is packed with vitamins A, K, & C, minerals such as iron, calcium, and magnesium, and has more antioxidants than most fruits or vegetables. Cilantro is a remarkable heavy-metal detoxifier and is able to remove mercury and aluminum from where it is stored in the adipose (fat) tissues. Cilantro is also able to mobilize mercury rapidly from the brain and central nervous system by separating it from the fat tissue and moving into the blood & lymph where when combined with a blue green algae such as spirulina it can be removed safely and effectively from the body. Cilantro & blue green algae used together is a winning combination and a natural miracle that has given tremendous relief to those suffering from mercury poisoning & toxicity. Cilantro also contains an anti-bacterial compound called dodecenal which has the ability to kill salmonella bacteria and prevent salmonella poisoning. Cilantro is highly beneficial for Alzheimer's disease, Parkinson's disease, Arthritis, Diabetes, Viral and Bacterial Infections, Hepatitis, Colitis, Obsessive-Compulsive Disorders, Autism, Tourette Syndrome, Infertility, and Bell's Palsy. Cilantro is also very helpful with autoimmune disorders such as Fibromyalgia, Addison's Disease, Guillain-Barre syndrome, IBS, Multiple Sclerosis, and Chronic Fatigue Syndrome. Cilantro is known to support the stomach, spleen, adrenals, thyroid, pancreas, bladder, and lungs. It is also highly beneficial in reducing LDL (bad) cholesterol and raising HDL (good) cholesterol. Cilantro is often juiced with celery and apples for a medicinal and healing drink. Juicing cilantro is one of the most effective ways to get at least one bunch or more of cilantro in you a day. Cilantro can also be added to smoothies, salsas, salads, guacamole, soups, pesto, tomatoes, beans, and veggie dishes. If the green flavor of cilantro does not appeal to you, yet you still want to receive its health benefits, consider using cilantro tincture or extract which can be found online or at your local health food store.

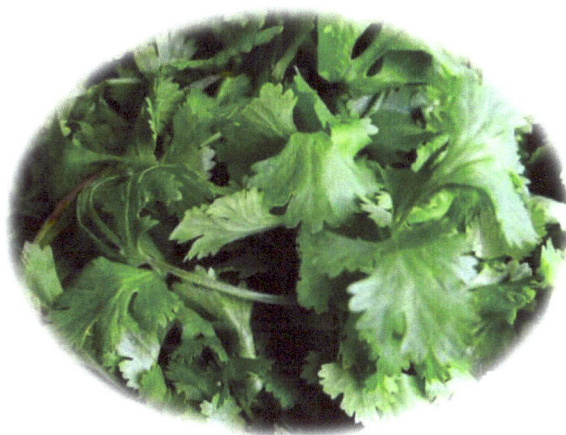

Smooth Skin
Winning The War On Ageing

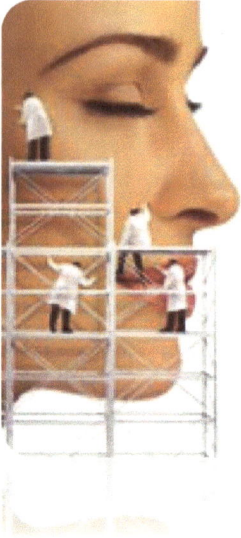

Fact:

- There are about 20 square feet of skin covering the average human body weighing 6 pounds.
- It takes 27 seconds for a product that is applied to the skin to enter the bloodstream.
- The entire epidermis is replaced approximately every 27 days.
- 98 percent of the atoms in the body are replaced yearly. Feed them life!

Most of us use 15 or more cosmetic and toiletry products each day according to the Seattle-based Toxic-Free Legacy Coalition.

Only 11% of these **chemicals** have been assessed for health and safety by any U.S. government agency, says the coalition, and one-third of all personal-care products contain at least one chemical linked to cancer. Some chemicals in these products also have links to birth defects and other health problems.

Chemicals in cosmetics that pose health risks, according to the Coalition, include suspected and proven carcinogens, endocrine disrupters, and neurotoxins.

Many problem ingredients do not appear on labels. Under current federal law, the cosmetics industry largely regulates itself. The U.S. Food and Drug Administration (FDA) does not require cosmetics manufacturers to have their products pre-approved before they are sold, to report cosmetics-related injuries or to file data on ingredients.

WRINKLING OF SKIN
(Dry Skin)

Wrinkles form when the skin loses its elasticity. As long as the skin is supple, any creasing of the skin disappears as soon as you stop making the expression that caused it. Over time these lines deepen into wrinkles. Some wrinkling is inevitable, as a result of aging. The first lines of wrinkles usually appear in the delicate tissue around the eyes-smile lines or "crow's feet." The cheeks and lips are next. As we age, our skin becomes both thinner and dryer, both of which contribute to the formation of wrinkles. Other factors include diet and nutrition, muscle tone, stress, proper skin care, exposure to environmental pollutants, and lifestyle habits such as smoking. Heredity also plays a role.

The most important factor of all is sun exposure, which not only dries out the skin but also leads to the generation of free radicals that can damage skin cells. It is estimated that as much as 90% of what we think of as signs of age are actually signs of overexposure. Overexposure is more than sunbathing or sunburn, approximately 70% of sun damage is incurred with everyday activities as driving and walking to and from your car. The sun effects are cumulative.

NUTRIENTS

Supplement	Suggested Dosage
	Very Important
Primrose oil	1,000 mg 3 times daily
Or	
Black currant seed oil	As directed on label
Vitamin A	25,000 IU daily for 3 months, then reduce to 15,000 daily
Natural carotenoid complex (Betatene)	As directed on label
Vitamin B complex	As directed on label
Vitamin B12	300-1,000 mg daily

Important

Kelp	1,000-1,500 mg daily
Selenium	200 mg daily
Silica	As directed on label
Vitamin C with bioflavonoids	3,000 mg daily in divided doses
Vitamin E	Start with 400IU daily, increase slowly to 800IU daily
Zinc	50 mg daily, do not exceed total of 100 mg daily from all supplements
Copper	3 mg daily

Helpful

Ageless Beauty from Biotec Foods	As directed on label
Aloe Vera	
Calcium and	1,500 mg daily
Magnesium	750 mg daily
Collagen cream	Apply topically as directed on label
Elastin cream	Apply topically as directed on label
Flaxseed oil capsules or Liquid	1,000 mg daily 1 tsp. Daily
Ultimate Oil from Nature's Secret	As directed on label
GH3 cream from Gero Vita	Apply topically as directed on label
Glucosamine sulfate or	As directed on label
N-Acetylglucosamine (NAG from Source Nat.)	As directed on label
Herpanacine from Diamond Herpanacine Assc.	As directed on label
Pycogenol	As directed on label
Super oxide dismutase (SOD)	As directed on label
Tretinoin (Retin-A)	As prescribed by physician
Vitamin D	400 IU daily

SKIN CARE

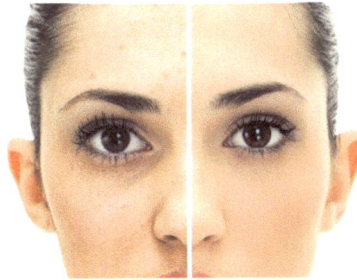

Acne is an inflammatory skin disorder that affects about 80% of all Americans between 12 and 24. It is more common in males. The sebaceous glands, located in each hair follicle or tiny pit of skin, produce oil that lubricates the skin. Sebaceous glands are fond in large numbers on the face, back chest and shoulders. Acne is not caused by "dirty pores", but more likely by overactive oil glands; the excess oil makes the pores sticky allowing bacteria to become trapped inside.

Blackheads form when sebum combines with skin pigments and plugs the pores. If scales below the surface of the skin become filled with sebum, whiteheads appear.

The exact cause of acne is not known, but factors that contribute to the condition include heredity, oily skin, and androgens. Other factors are allergies; stress; the use of certain drugs (especially steroids, lithium); over consumption of junk food, saturated fats, hydrogenated fats and animal product; nutritional deficiencies; exposure to industrial pollutants; and over washing or repeated rubbing of the skin.

The skin also "breathes". If the pores become clogged the microbes that are involved in causing acne flourish because they are protected against the bacteriostatic action of sunshine. Dust, dirt, oils and grime from pollution clog the pores, but this can be eliminated by washing the skin properly. A body ph that is too high or too alkaline, also fosters the nesting and breeding of acne-causing bacteria.

Nutrients

Supplement	Suggested Dosage
Very important	
Chromium picolinate	As directed on label
Essential fatty acids (flaxseed oil or primrose oil)	As directed on label
Vitamin B complex	100mg 3 times daily
Extra vitamin b3 (niacin)	100 mg 3 times daily
Pantothenic acid (vitamin B5)	50 mg 3 times daily
Vitamin B6 (pyridoxine)	50 mg 3 times daily
Zinc	30-80mg daily-Do not exceed a total of 100mg from all supplements

Colloidal silver	Take orally or apply topically as directed on label
Garlic (Kyolic)	2 capsules 3 times daily, with meals
Potassium	99 mg daily
Vitamin A	25,000 IU daily until healed, then reduce to 5,000 IU daily
Natural carotenoid complex (Betatene)	As directed on label
Vitamin E	400 IU daily

Helpful

Acidophilus	As directed on label-Take on empty stomach
Chlorophyll	As directed on label
GH3 cream from Gero Vita	Apply topically as directed on label
Herpanacine from Diamond-Herpanacine	As directed on label
Multienzyme complex with hydrochloric acid	As directed on label. Take with meals
L-Cysteine	500mg daily, on an empty stomach. Take with juice Or water, not with milk. Take with 50mg vitamin B6 and 100 mg vitamin C for better absorption.
Lecithin granules	1 tbsp 3 times daily before meals
Or capsules	1,200 mg 3 times daily, before meals
Proteolytic enzymes	As directed on label-take with and between meals
Selenium	200 mg daily
Shark cartilage (Benefin)	1gm per 15 lbs of body weight daily, divided by 3 doses.
Tretinoin (Retin-A)	As prescribed by physician
Vitamin C with bioflavonoids	3,000-5,000 mg daily in divided doses
Vitamin D	400 IU daily

HERBS

Burdock root and red clover are powerful blood cleansers.

A poultice using chaparral, dandelion and yellow dock root can be applied directly to the acne areas

Unless the area is extensive or badly inflamed, you may use a steam treatment of lavender, red clover, and strawberry leaves. Simmer a total of 2-4 tablespoons of herbs in 2 quarts of water, when steaming; sit with your face a comfortable distance over the steam for 15 min. Then splash with cold water and allow skin to air dry

Tea tree oil is a natural antibiotic and antiseptic. Dab full-strength (sparingly) 3 times per day or add 1 dropper full of the oil to ¼ cup warm water and pat on affected area with a 100% cotton clean ball. Tea tree oil soap also works well

Other beneficial herbs include alfalfa, cayenne, dandelion root, Echinacea and yellow dock root.

RECOMMENDATIONS

Eat a high fiber diet. Increase your intake of raw foods with oxalic acid, including almonds, beets, cashews, and Swiss chard. Exceptions are spinach and rhubarb, which should be consumed only in small amounts.

Eat more foods rich in zinc, including shellfish, soybeans, whole grains, sunflower seeds, and a small amount of nuts daily. Eat plenty of soured products, such as low-fat yogurt. Avoid alcohol, butter, caffeine, cheese, chocolate, cocoa, cream, eggs, fat, fish, fried foods, hot and spicy foods, hydrogenated oils and shortenings, margarine, meat, poultry, wheat, soft drinks, and foods containing brominated vegetable oil. Try eliminating dairy products from your diet for 1 month. Avoid all forms of sugar, eliminate all processed foods from the diet and do not use iodized salt. Keep the affected area as free of oil as possible. Shampoo your hair frequently. Use an all-natural soap with sulfur designed for acne (available at health food stores). Wash your skin thoroughly, but gently; never rub hard. Avoid wearing make-up. Friction makes pimples more likely to rupture, so avoid wearing tight clothing like turtlenecks. If you shave, use a standard blade, not an electric razor and always shave in the direction of hair growth. Try to avoid stress, exercise, get 15 min. of sunshine each day and get a sufficient amount of sleep. Avoid oral or topical steroids, and do squeeze the spots. Don't touch the affected area unless your hands are thoroughly clean.

CONSIDERATIONS

For severe acne, the drug isotretinoin is the only reliable treatment. The best weapon for moderate cases is topical tretinoin (Retin-A). An antibiotic cream or an oral antibiotic is sometimes prescribed. Long-term use of antibiotics,often leads to candida infection. If you take antibiotics, use some form of acidophilus. Benzoyl peroxide is the active ingredient in most over-the-counter products, don't apply around eyes and mouth. Blackheads should not be squeezed, but removed with a specially designed instrument to avoid scarring. Niacinamide, kombucha tea,dimethylsulfoxide(only from a health food store, not the commercial kind found in hardware stores), and a treatment program called Derma-Klear from Enzymatic Therapy are all good products.

OILY SKIN

Oily skin occurs when the sebaceous (oil-secreting) glands produce more oil than is needed for proper lubrication of the skin. This excess oil can clog pores and cause blemishes. Oily skin is probably largely a matter of heredity, but it is known to be affected by factors such as diet, hormone levels, pregnancy, birth control pills, and cosmetics you use. Humidity and hot weather also stimulate the sebaceous glands to produce more oil. Because skin tends to become dryer with age, and because of the hormonal shifts of adolescence, oily skin is common in teenagers, but it can occur at any age. Many people have skin that is oily only in certain areas and dry or normal in others, a condition known as combination skin. In general, the forehead, nose, chin, and upper back tend to be oilier than other areas.

Oily skin has its positive aspects. It is slow to develop age spots and discoloration, fine lines, and wrinkles. It often doesn't freckle or turn red in the sun-on the contrary, it tans evenly and beautifully. On the negative side, oily skin is prone to "breakouts" well past adolescence and has a chronically shiny appearance, an oily or greasy feeling, and enlarged pores.

Unless otherwise specified, the dosages recommended here are for adults. For a child between the ages of twelve and seventeen, reduce the dose to three-quarters of the recommended amount.

NUTRIENTS

SUPPLEMENT	SUGGESTED DOSAGE	COMMENTS
Very Important		
Flaxseed oil capsules	1,000 mg daily.	Supplies needed essential
Or		fatty acids. A good healer
Liquid	1 tsp daily.	For most skin disorders.
Or		
Primrose oil	Up to 500 mg daily.	Contains linoeic acid, which is needed by the skin.
Vitamin A	25,000 IU daily for	Necessary for healing and
With	3 months then reduce	construction of new skin
Mixed carotenoids	to 15,000 IU daily. If You are pregnant, do not exceed 10,000 IU daily.	tissue.

Vitamin B complex Plus extra Vitamin B12	As directed on label. 1,000-2,000 mcg daily.	B vitamins are important for healthy skin tone.
Important Kelp	1,000-1,500 mcg daily.	Supplies balanced minerals Needed for good skin tone.
Vitamin E	Start with 400 IU daily And increase slowly 800 IU daily.	Protects against free radicals. Use d-alpha-tocopherol form.
Zinc Plus Copper	50 mg daily. Do not Exceeded a total of 100 mg Daily from all supplements. 3 mg daily.	For tissue repair. Enhances immune response. Use zinc Gluconate lozenges or optiZinc for best absorption. Needed to balance with zinc.
Helpful GH3 cream From Gero Vita	Apply topically as directed on label.	Good for acne. Also good for any discoloration of the skin.
Grape seed extract	As directed on label.	A powerful antioxidant that Protects skin cells.
Herpanacine from Diamond-Herpanacine Associates	As directed on label.	Contains antioxidants, amino acids, and herbs that promote overall skin health.
L-Cysteine	500 mg daily, on an Empty stomach. Take With water or juice. Do Not take with milk. Take With 50 mg vitamin B6 And 100 mg vitamin C For better absorption.	Contains sulfur, needed for healthy skin.
Lecithin granules Or Capsules	1 tbsp 3 times daily, before meals. 1,200 mg 3 times daily, Before meals.	Needed for better absorption Of essential fatty acids.
Superoxide Dismutase (SOD)	As directed on label.	Free radical destroyer.
Tretinoin (Retin-A)	As prescribed by Physician.	Acts as gradual chemical Peel; unclogs pores and speeds Up sloughing off of top layers Of skin, exposing new, fresh Skin. Available by prescription only.

HERBS

- Aloe Vera has excellent healing properties. Apply aloe vera gel topically, as directed on product label or as needed.
- Burdock root, chamomile, horsetail, oat straw, and thymes nourish the skin.
- Lavender is very good for oily skin. Mist your skin with lavender water several times daily.
- A facial sauna using lemongrass, licorice root, and rosebuds is good for oily skin. Two or three times a week, simmer a total of 2 to 4 tablespoons of dried or fresh herbs in 2 quarts of water. When the pot is steaming, place it on top of a trivet or thick potholder on a table, and sit with your face at a comfortable distance over the steam for fifteen minutes. You can use a towel to trap the steam if you wish. After fifteen minutes, splash your face with cold water and allow your skin to air dry or pat it dry with a towel. After the sauna, you can allow the herbal water to cool and save it for use as a toning lotion to be dabbed on your face with a cotton ball after cleansing.
- Try a steam facial using the herbal laxative Swiss Kriss twice a week to remove excess oils from the skin. Add about 2 tablespoons per two quarts of water.
- Witch hazel applied to the skin is excellent for absorbing oil.

RECOMMENDATIONS

- Drink plenty of quality water to keep the skin hydrated and flush out toxins.

- Reduce the amount of fat in your diet. Consume no fried foods, animal fats, or heat-processed vegetable oils such as those sold in supermarkets. Do not cook with oil, and do not eat any oils that have been subjected to heat, whether in processing or cooking. If a little oil is necessary, such as in salad dressing, use cold-pressed canola or olive oil only.

- Do not drink soft drinks or alcoholic beverages. Avoid sugar, chocolate, and junk food.

- Keep your skin very clean. Wash your face two or three times in the course of a day- no more, because too much washing will stimulate your skin to produce more oil. Use your hands instead of harsh scrubs or washcloths. Sterile gauze pads are also good for cleaning the skin. (Do not use a pad more than once.) Do not use harsh soaps or cleansers. Use a pure soap with no artificial additives, such as E Gem Skin Care Soap from Carlson Laboratories. Do not use cleansers or lotions that contain alcohol. After cleansing, apply a natural *oil-free* moisturizer to keep the skin supple.

- Use hot water when washing your face. Hot water dissolves skin oil better than lukewarm or cold water.

- Try using a clay or mud mask. White or rose-colored clays are best for sensitive skin.

- Choose cosmetic and facial care products specifically designed for oily skin.

- Alpha-hydroxy acids are a group of naturally occurring acids (found mostly in fruits) that help to stimulate cell renewal, aid the skin in retaining water, and give it a smoother, less oily appearance. Oily skin can benefit from the use of products containing alpha-hydroxy acids because they aid in removal of the top layer of dead skin cells, which stimulates healthy skin growth and may diminish large pores. Glycolic acid is probably the best of the alpha-hydroxy acids for this purpose. If you decide to try an alpha-hydroxy acid product, begin with a product containing 5 percent alpha-hydroxy acid (not more), and apply it at night only. First wash your face, then wait five minutes before applying a small amount of the product. After two or three weeks of nighttime application, you can begin applying the product in the morning as well. As your skin becomes accustomed to the effects of alpha-hydroxy acids, you may wish to work your way up to higher-concentration products.

- Products containing benzoyl peroxide are effective for oily skin. Start with a mild-strength formula to minimize possible irritation.

- Choose an astringent that contains acetone, which is known for dissolving oil.

- To clear away excess oil, use a clay or mud mask. Blend together well 1 teaspoon green clay powder (available in health food stores) and 1 teaspoon raw honey. Apply mixture to your face, avoiding the eye area. Leave it on for 15 minutes, then rinse well with lukewarm water. Do this at least 3 times a week-or more often if necessary. White or rose-colored clays are best for sensitive skin.

- Once or twice daily, mix equal parts of lemon juice and water together. Pat mixture on your face and allow it to dry, then rinse with warm water. Follow with a cool-water rinse.

- Look for facial powder that contains talcum powder. It is oil-free and blots the oil on your skin.

- For combination skin, simply treat the oily areas as oily skin and the dry areas as dry skin.

- Do not smoke. Smoking promotes enlargement of the pores and impairs the overall health of the skin.

CONSIDERATIONS

- Caring for oily skin does not mean trying to dry the skin out. Despite having excess oil, skin may still lack moisture. Moisture is a term that is used to refer to the amount of water inside the skin cells, not the amount of oil on the surface of the skin. While oil and moisture levels are related (the oil helps prevent loss of moisture through evaporation), the two are not the same. There are products available that help to supply and protect moisture without adding oil. Vitamin A Moisturizing Gel from Derma-E Products is a good nongreasy moisturizer. Using such a moisturizer may help prevent the development of wrinkles in the long run.

- Many companies that specialize in skin care have developed foil-wrapped packets of wipes saturated in alcohol for skin care away from home. These can be placed in your briefcase or purse for cutting through the oil and freshening up the skin.

- Although it is a common myth, oily skin doesn't actually cause acne. Although there is an association between the severity of acne and the amount of oil a person's skin produces, not all people with oily skin have acne.

This incredible detox drink helps you burn fat, boost metabolism, lose weight, fight diabetes and lower blood pressure.

Ingredients

1 glass of water (12-16 oz.)
2 Tbsp. Apple Cider Vinegar
2 Tbsp. lemon juice
1 tsp. cinnamon
1 Tbsp. Raw Honey

Directions
Blend all ingredients together

Secret Recipe Detox Drink will help your body burn fat, lose weight, fight diabetes.

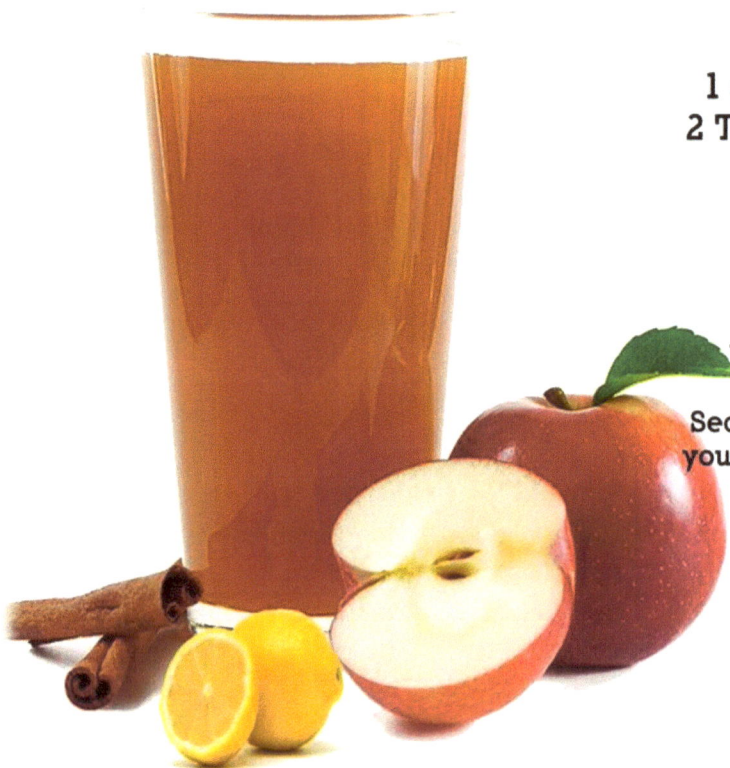

Living With Crohn's Disease

Crohn's disease is an inflammatory bowel disorder of unknown origin. It usually affects the lowest portion of the small intestine, but it can occur in other parts of the digestive tract, from the mouth to the anus. Crohn's disease causes inflammation that extends deep into the lining of the intestinal wall, frequently causing crampy abdominal pain, diarrhea, rectal bleeding, loss of appetite, and weight loss. A common complication of the disease is blockage of the intestine caused by scar tissue that narrows the passageway. The disease may also cause sores, or ulcers, that break through to the surrounding tissues. People with Crohn's disease also suffer from nutritional deficiencies.

A relatively small percentage of people (1.2 to 15 cases per 100,000 people in the United States) is affected by Crohn's disease. It affects men and women equally and tends to run in families. According to the Crohn's and Colitis Foundation of America (CCFA), people who have a relative with the disease have at least ten times the risk of developing Crohn's disease compared with the general population. This disorder affects people in all age groups, but the onset usually occurs either between ages fifteen and thirty or between ages sixty and eighty. Children with Crohn's disease may suffer delayed development and stunted growth due to nutritional deficiencies.

Crohn's disease can be difficult to diagnose because its symptoms are similar to those of other intestinal disorders, particularly ulcerative colitis-another inflammatory which affects only the colon. Crohn's symptoms can also appear intermittently, occurring every few months to every few years for some people. In rare cases, the symptoms may appear once or twice and not return. If the disease continues for many years, bowel function gradually deteriorates. Left untreated it can become extremely serious, even life threatening, and it may increase the risk of cancer by as much as twenty times.

Doctors believe that Crohn's disease has a genetic basis, but that it does not appear until triggered by the presence of bacteria or virus that provokes an abnormal activation of the immune system. The onset of Crohn's disease can be dramatic, with alarming symptoms such as sudden high fever, sudden weight loss of more than five pounds in a few days, rectal bleeding, severe abdominal pain that persists for more than an hour at a time, and persistent vomiting accompanied by a cessation of bowel movements. A series of tests may be required to confirm Crohn's disease. Blood tests may be done to check for anemia and/or a high white blood count. A doctor do an upper gastrointestinal x-ray series to look at the small intestine, or a colonoscopy, in which the doctor inspects the interior of the large intestine using a long, flexible lighted tube linked to a computer and monitor. If the tests show the presence of Crohn's disease, the doctor may do more x-rays of both the upper and lower digestive tract to find out how much is affected by the disease.

Since there is no cure for Crohn's disease, the goals of treatment are to control inflammation, relive symptoms, and correct nutritional deficiencies- all of which can help keep Crohn's disease in remission.
Unless otherwise specified, the dosages recommended here are for adults. For a child between the ages of twelve and seventeen, reduce the dose to three-quarters of the recommended amount. For a child between six and twelve, use one-half of the recommended dose, and for a child under the age of six, use one-quarter of the recommended amount.

SUPPLEMENT	SUGGESTED DOSAGE	COMMENTS
ESSENTIAL		
Duodenal glandular	As directed on label.	Acids in healing gastrointestinal ulcers.
L-Glutamine	500mg twice daily, on an empty stomach. Take with water or juice. Do not take with milk. Take with 50mg vitamin B6 and 100mg vitamin C for better absorption.	A major metabolic fuel for the intestinal cells; maintains the villi, the absorption surfaces of the gut.
Liver extract Injections Plus	2cc once weekly or as prescribed by physician.	Needed for proper digestion.
Vitamin B complex and	1cc once weekly or as prescribed by physician.	Helps to prevent anemia.
vitamin B12 and	1cc twice weekly or as prescribed by physician.	Important for proper digestion and to prevent anemia. Deficiency aggravates mal-absorption.
folic acid	1/4cc twice weekly or as prescribed by physician.	needed for constant supply of new cells. Injections (under a doctors supervision) are best.
or vitamin B complex	100mg 3 times daily.	If injections are not available, use lozenge or sublingual form.
plus extra vitamin B12 and	1,000-2,000 mg daily.	
folic acid	200 mcg daily.	
N-Acetylglucosamine (N-A-G from Source Naturals)	As directed on label.	A major constituent of the barrier layer that protects the intestinal lining from digestive enzymes and other potentially damaging intestinal contents.

Omega-3 essential Fatty acids (Kyolic-EPA from Wakunaga, Intestamend from Health From the Sun, Flaxseed oil, primrose Oil, and salmon oil Are good sources)	As directed on label.	Needed for repair of the digestive tract; reduces inflammatory processes. Studies show essential fatty acids may reduce Crohn's symptoms and aid in maintaining remission.
Pancreatin Plus Bromelain	As directed on label. Take with meals. As directed on label.	To break down protein and Assist digestion.
Taurine Plus from American Biologics	500 mg daily, on an empty stomach. Take With 50 mg vitamin B6 And 100 mg vitamin C For better absorption.	An important antioxidant and immune regulator. Use the sublingual form.
Vitamin C With Bioflavonoids	1,000 mg 3 times daily.	Prevents inflammation and improves immunity. Use buffered type.
Vitamin K	As directed on label.	Vital to colon health. Deficiency is common in people with this disorder due to malabsorption and diarrhea.
Zinc	50 mg daily. Do not Exceed a total of 100 mg daily from All supplements.	Needed for the immune system and for healing. Use zinc gluconate lozenges or OptiZinc for best absorption.
IMPORTANT Free-form amino Acid complex (Amino Balance From Anabol Naturals)	¼ tsp twice daily.	Protein is essential in the healing of the intestine. use a sublingual form.
Garlic (Kyolic)	2 capsules 3 times Daily, with meals.	Combats free radicals in Crohn's disease. Acids healing.
Lactobacilli (Kyo-Dophilus From Wakunaga) Or	As directed on label.	Aids in digestion. Use a nondairy formula. A product containing both L. Acidophilus and L. Bifidus is best.

Capricin from Probiologic	As directed on label.	works in conjunction with butyric acid to reduce inflammation and seepage of undigested food particles.
Spiru-tein from Nature's Plus	2 capsules 3 times daily.	Supplies necessary protein. Helps stabilize blood sugar between meals.

HELPFUL

Calcium And Magnesium	2,000 mg daily. 1,500 mg daily.	Aids in preventing colon cancer.
Floradix Iron + Herbs from Salus Haus	2 tsp daily.	To prevent anemia. Floradix is a readily absorbable form of iron that is nontoxic and derived from food sources.
Gastro-Calm from Olympain Labs	As directed on label.	A combination of herbs and digestive enzymes to help relieve indigestion and reduce gastrointestinal inflammation.
Multivitamin and Mineral complex With Copper And Manganese And Selenium Plus extra Potassium	As directed on label. 99 mg daily.	Mal-absorption is often a result of this disorder. Copper, selenium, and manganese are important for treating this disorder and are often deficient because of absorption problems. Use a liquid, powder, or a capsule formula. May reduce surgical Complications and also The need for surgery.
Oxy-Caps from Earth's Bounty	As directed on label.	An oxygen supplement to counter nutritional deficiencies caused by Crohn's disease.

Quercetin	500 mg twice daily, Before meals.	Slows histamine release; helps control food allergies. Needed for a variety of enzyme functions.
Plus Bromelain or Activated Quercetin From Source Naturals	100 mg twice daily, before meals. As directed on label.	Improves absorption of Quercetin. Contains quercetin plus bromelain and vitamin C.
Shark cartilage (BeneFin)	As directed on label. If you cannot tolerate taking It orally, it can be Administered rectally In a retention enema.	Fights metastasis of cancerous tumors.
Vitamin A And Vitamin E	25,000 IU daily. If you Are pregnant, do not exceed 10,000 IU daily. Up to 800 IU daily.	Antioxidants that aid in controlling infection and in repair of the intestinal tract. use emulsion forms for easier assimilation . Use d-alpha-tocopherol form of Vitamin E.
Vitamin D3	400 IU daily.	Prevents metabolic bone disease from developing as a result of mal-absorption.

HERBS

- Aloe vera is beneficial for Crohn's disease because it softens stools and has a healing effect on the digestive tract. Drink ½ cup of aloe vera juice three times daily.

- There are many combination herbal products designed to offer gastrointestinal relief. Enzymatic Therapy, Olympain Labs, and Solaray are recommended sources.

- Other herbs that are good for this disorder include burdock root, Echinacea, fenugreek, goldenseal, licorice, marshmallow root, pau d' arco, enteric-coated peppermint (do not use any other form), red clover, rose hips, silymarin (milk thistle extract), slippery elm, and yerba maté. These herbs support digestion, cleanse the bloodstream, and reduce inflammation and infection. For best results, use them on an alternating basis.

- *CAUTION:* Do not use licorice on a daily basis for more than seven days in a row, and avoid it completely if you have high blood pressure. Do not take goldenseal on a daily basis for more than one week at a time, and do not use it during pregnancy. If you have a history of cardiovascular disease, diabetes, or glaucoma, use it only under a doctor's supervision.

RECOMMENDATIONS

- Eat a diet consisting mainly of non-acidic fresh or cooked vegetables such as broccoli, Brussels sprouts, cabbage, carrots, celery, garlic, kale, spinach, and turnips. Steam, broil, boil, or bake your food.

- Drink plenty of liquids, such as steam-distilled water, herbal teas, and fresh juices. Fresh cabbage juice is very beneficial.

- Add papaya to your diet. Chew a couple of the seeds to aid digestion.

- During an acute attack, eat organic baby foods, steamed vegetables, and well-cooked brown rice, millet, and oatmeal.

- Try eliminating all dairy foods (including cheese), fish, hard sausage, pickled cabbage, and yeast products from your diet, and see if symptoms improve. These foods are high in histamine. Many people with Crohn's disease are histamine-intolerant. Milk and other dairy products also contain carrageenan, a compound extracted from red seaweed. Carrageenan, which is widely used in the food industry for its ability to stabilize milk proteins, has been shown to induce ulcerative colitis in laboratory animals.

- Avoid alcohol, caffeine, carbonated beverages, chocolate, corn, nuts, popcorn, eggs, foods with artificial additives or preservatives, fried and greasy foods, margarine, meat, dairy products such as milk and cheese, pepper, spicy foods, tobacco, white flour, and all animal products, with the exception of white fish from clear waters. These foods are irritating to the digestive tract. Mucus-forming foods such as processed refined foods and dairy products should also be avoided. Limit your intake of barley, rye, and wheat.

- Avoid refined carbohydrates. Do not consume such foods as boxed dry cereals or anything containing any form of sugar. Diets high in refined carbohydrates have been associated with Crohn's disease. These foods must be eliminated from the diet.

- Check stools daily for bleeding.

- As much as possible, avoid stress. Our thoughts, nervous systems, and bodily functions are deeply interconnected. Our thoughts and moods affect our bodies. During an attack, rest is important.

- Make sure the bowels move daily, but do not use harsh laxatives. Gentle enemas made by adding a dropperful of alcohol-free herbal extract and 1 teaspoon of nondairy acidophilus powder to 2 quarts of lukewarm water are good. Accumulations of toxic body wastes often become breeding grounds for parasitic infestation. Toxins can also be absorbed into the bloodstream through the colon wall. Psyllium husks should be used daily for fiber; this aids in removing toxins before they are absorbed.
  NOTE: Always take supplemental fiber separately from other supplements and medications.

- Do not use rectal suppositories that contain hydrogenated chemically prepared fats.

- If you are constipated, use a cleansing enema.

- Use a heating pad to reduce abdominal pain.

CONSIDERATIONS

- There are no consistent dietary rules that apply to everyone, but people with Crohn's disease are generally encouraged to eat a healthy diet to help the body replace lost nutrients. Moreover, some nutrients, such as essential fatty acids and the amino acid glutamine, have been shown to help maintain a state of remission.

- It is important that nutritional deficiencies be corrected for healing. Persons with inflammatory bowel disorders require as much as 30 percent more protein than normal. If chronic diarrhea is present, electrolyte and trace mineral deficiencies should be considered. Chronic steatorrhea (fatty stools resulting from improper digestion of fats) may results in deficiencies of calcium and magnesium.

- Drugs such as corticosteroids and sulfasalazine (Azulfidine), which are prescribed for inflammatory bowel diseases, and cholestyramine (Questran), which is prescribed to lower cholesterol levels, increase the need for nutritional supplements. Corticosteroids depress protein synthesis and inhibit normal calcium absorption by increasing excretion of vitamin C in the urine. Deficiencies of other nutrients, such as zinc, potassium, vitamin B6 (pyridoxine), folic acid, and vitamin D, decrease bone formation and slow healing. Sulfasalazine inhibits the transport of folic acid and iron, causing anemia.

- Antioxidants have been shown to increase the risk of developing Crohn's disease. The intestinal walls normally contain small amounts of the antioxidant enzymes superoxide dismutase (SOD), catalase, and glutathione peroxidase, but their ability to fight free radicals may be overwhelmed during periods of active inflammation, resulting in tissue damage.

- To reestablish a proper healing environment, it is necessary to maintain a generally alkaline bodily pH.

- Adhering to an allergen-free diet, replacing lost nutrients, and using selected herbs can speed healing and may prevent future disturbances. Studies have proven that when a person who has achieved remission goes back to his or her former diet, Crohn's disease returns. Other things that have trauma, and psychosomatic and vascular factors.

- Nutritional deficiencies resulting from malabsorption may weaken the immune system, in turn prolonging the time required for the inflammation and ulcers to heal.

- Many microorganisms have been considered as possible causes of Crohn's disease, including fungi, bacteria, viruses, mycobacteria, pseudomonas-like organisms, and Chlamydia. However, the cause of Crohn's disease has not yet been established. It is likely that multiple factors are involved.

- Antigenic reactions may result from "leaky gut syndrome," in which minute particles of undigested or partially digested food pass through the swollen and inflamed mucosal wall into the bloodstream, where they cause reactions. The mucosal wall must be repaired to avoid this. Avoiding foods that cause a reaction is important. Treatment with butyric acid, a monounsaturated fatty acid, reduces inflammatory conditions, reduces seepage of undigested food particles, and aids in repair of the mucosal wall. N-acetylglucosamine (NAG) prevents leaky gut syndrome.

- A study done in Italy found that people with Crohn's disease who took sustained-release fish oil supplements were less likely to suffer relapses than those who did not. Of the subjects in the one year study who took fish oil, over half remained symptom-free, compared with only a quarter of those who took a placebo.

- Researchers have not been able to find a specific genetic marker for Crohn's disease, but they have found that the illness is four times more common in Caucasians and Jewish people than in people of other ethnic backgrounds. In 20 to 40 percent of reported cases, multiple family members have suffered either from Crohn's disease or ulcerative colitis.

- Most people with Crohn's disease are initially treated with drugs such as corticosteroids to help control inflammation. Drugs that suppress the immune system are also used, but they can increase susceptibility to infection. The Food and Drug Administration (FDA) has now approved a genetically engineered product called infliximab (Remicade) for people with moderate-to-severe Crohn's disease who have not responded to traditional treatments. Remicade is made from human and mouse cells, and works specifically against a protein that promotes inflammation in the body. In drug trials, one dose relieved many of the symptoms for two to four weeks, after which the benefits waned. Scientists are still studying the long-term effects.

- If Crohn's disease continues for many years, bowel function gradually deteriorates. Surgery may be required to remove the diseased portion of the intestine. While this surgery does not cure the disease, it can relieve symptoms, and five years later at least 50 percent of people who undergo it are in good health, can work full time, and enjoy life without being restricted by diarrhea or pain.

- People with Crohn's disease have a significantly higher than normal risk of developing colon cancer. If you have this disorder, you should undergo a colonoscopy at least once every two years, starting eight to ten years after diagnosis.

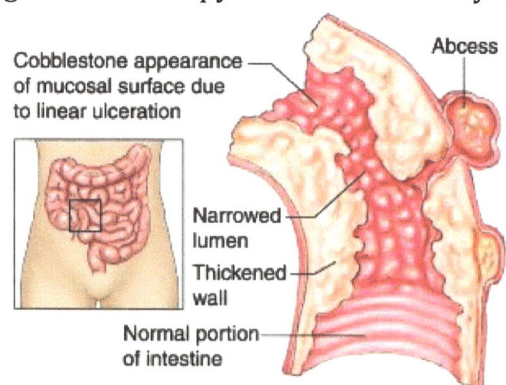

Cobblestone appearance of mucosal surface due to linear ulceration

Abcess

Narrowed lumen

Thickened wall

Normal portion of intestine

Did you know 1 clove of raw garlic contains as much antibiotics as about a hundred thousand units of penicillin?

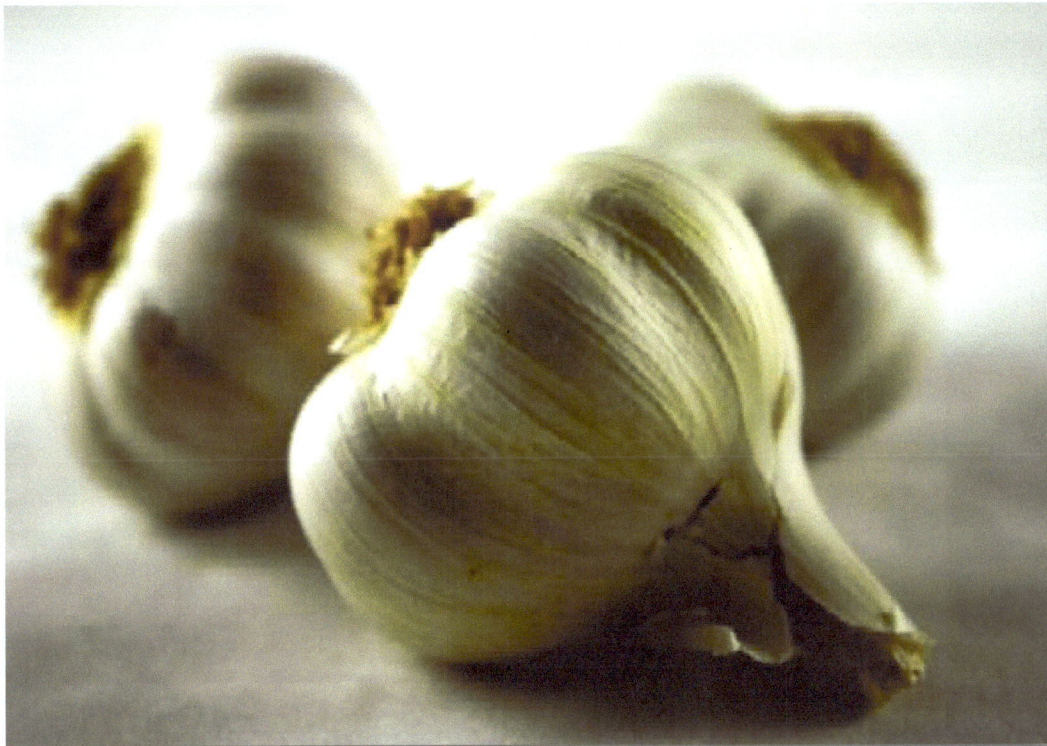

Living Water

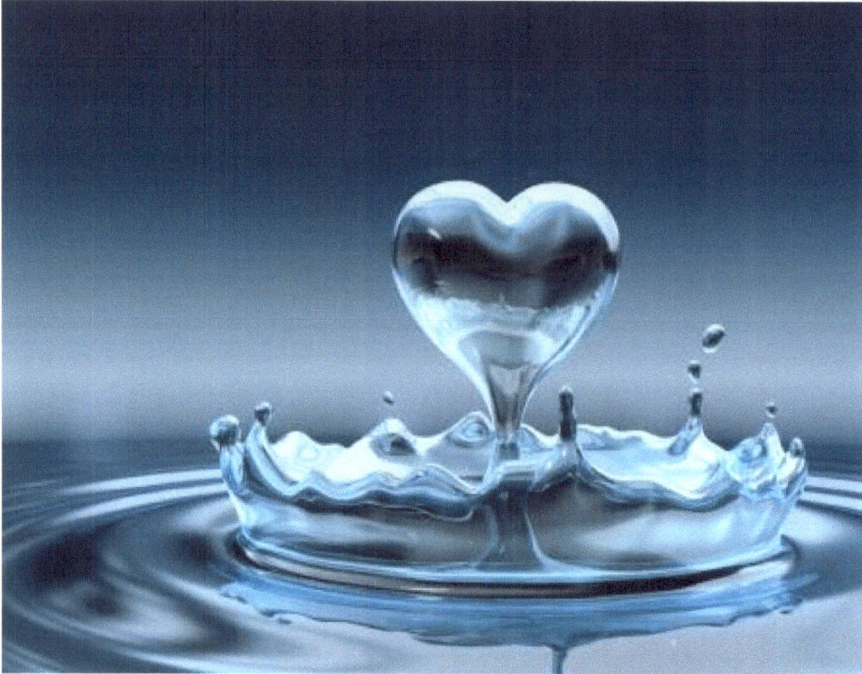

Water is life's matter and matrix, mother and medium. There is no life without water.

Alkaline drinking water is gaining in recognition and popularity among alternative health professionals and consumers alike. It is accepted in ever widening circles that an alkalizing diet may have a positive impact on health and vitality. The mild alkalinity of Advanced Hydration Technology makes it an excellent choice as one component of a diet designed to support optimum pH levels in the body. Here is why. The pH scale ranges from 0, on the acidic end, to 14 on the alkaline end with 7 being neutral. Many people erroneously assume all drinking water is neutral. The fact is, distilled water is neutral, while much of the drinking water available to us, whether from the tap or bottled, is acidic. Have you ever noticed that when you are not thirsty even bottled water doesn't taste very good and has an after taste? That after taste can be caused by chemicals (chlorine, fluoride), certain types of minerals or other dissolved solids in the water creating acidity.

Advanced Hydration Technology alkaline drinking water is slightly alkaline on the pH scale. This mild level of alkalinity is perfect to help maintain the 7.35 - 7.45 average pH level that is optimum for your blood. There are two primary reasons why it is important to address your blood's pH. First, pH is a factor that has a critical effect on your blood's capacity to uptake, carry and deliver oxygen to all parts of your body. Blood pH is highest just after it leaves your lungs, around 7.6, and lowest just before it returns to your lungs at 7.3 or a little less.

Along its journey, as your blood begins to give up oxygen, carbon dioxide (CO_2) molecules replace the lost oxygen in the red blood cells. The CO_2 represents acidic waste that will be released either in the kidneys or the lungs for elimination. When oxygen is lost and replaced by CO_2 in the red blood cells, the alkalinity of your blood decreases. As alkalinity decreases it becomes more difficult for the red blood cells to hold the remaining oxygen, or, to put it another way, it becomes easier for your blood to release oxygen to your body. There is a delicate balance between CO_2 and alkalinity that must be maintained to ensure oxygen is effectively distributed. Second, your blood is the primary regulator of pH levels in all parts of your body. If your blood's pH is lower than it should be, it loses its effectiveness in this function. One function of oxygen in the metabolic process is to convert cellular waste into CO_2 so it can be removed by the blood. A lower pH means blood is leaving your lungs with less oxygen, delivering less oxygen and eliminating waste less efficiently. The resulting buildup of non-disposed waste in the fluid between cells creates an acidic, low oxygen environment that anaerobic pathogens thrive in. Some strains of cancer prefer this type of environment as well as a number of pathogenic bacteria. Low pH and low oxygen can be a symptom of other health problems or it can become a chronic condition called Acid Hypoxia that results from years of poor health and dietary habits.

Advanced Hydration Technology helps maintain your blood's optimum pH which, in turn, will help balance the necessary conditions for your blood to carry a maximum load of oxygen, and support your blood's capacity to properly regulate pH levels in all parts of your body. Unfortunately, for many of us, our lifestyles and dietary habits have a negative effect on our pH balance. This can directly influence our immediate health and vitality as well as create cumulative effects that will negatively affect our long-term health. For example, there are two characteristics of this country's most popular beverages, soft drinks and coffee that make it difficult for you to maintain your optimum pH balance.

First, they are caffeinated and/or artificially sweetened, which makes them diuretic- the fluid lost because of these beverages can actually exceed what the beverage provides. Consequently, many people are unknowingly in a mild state of undiagnosed dehydration.

Second, these beverages are also very acidic. Because the waste produced by your metabolism is already acidic, the consumption of large amounts of acidic beverages creates even more downward pressure on your pH. Add to this the fact that a lack of aerobic exercise has resulted, for many people, in diminished cardio-pulmonary capacity. Mild dehydration, excessive consumption of acidic beverages and diminished cardio-pulmonary capacity translates into not enough water and oxygen to efficiently convert energy and eliminate waste.

Is it any wonder we need stimulants in our beverages to get through the day? The acidic pressure on our pH balance is tremendous! Perhaps it's time to make a change in the water you drink. We can't live without it so why not drink water that tastes great all the time and has some unique, helpful characteristics as well. For those who like to drink cold water, this article is applicable to you. It is nice to have a cup of cold drink after a meal. However, the cold water will solidify the oily stuff that you have just consumed. It will slow down the digestion. Once this 'sludge' reacts with the acid, it will break down and be absorbed by the intestine faster than the solid food. It will line the **intestine**. Very soon, this will turn into fats and lead to cancer. It is best to drink hot soup or warm water after a meal.

A serious note about heart attacks, You should know that not every heart attack symptom is going to be the left arm hurting. Be aware of intense pain in the jaw line. You may never have the first chest pain during the course of a heart attack. Nausea and intense sweating are also common symptoms. 60% of people who have a heart attack while they are asleep do not wake up. Pain in the jaw can wake you from a sound sleep. Let's be careful and be aware. The more we know, the better chance we could survive.

Gross Anatomy of the Heart Anterior view

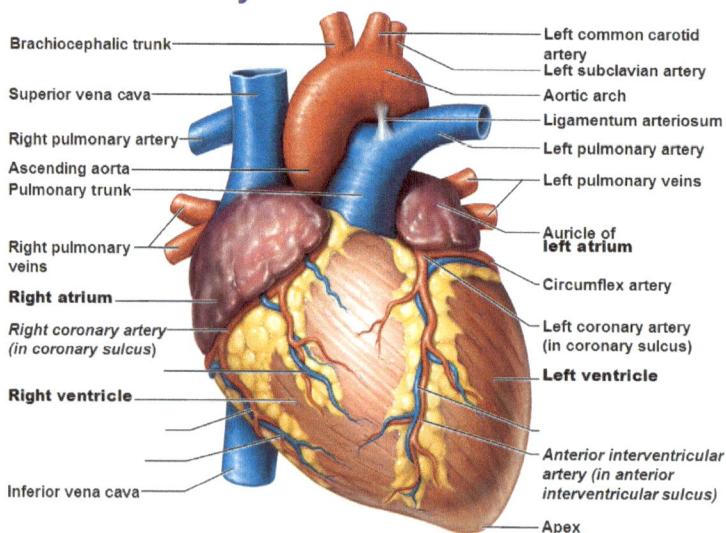

Brachiocephalic trunk
Superior vena cava
Right pulmonary artery
Ascending aorta
Pulmonary trunk
Right pulmonary veins
Right atrium
Right coronary artery (in coronary sulcus)
Right ventricle
Inferior vena cava

Left common carotid artery
Left subclavian artery
Aortic arch
Ligamentum arteriosum
Left pulmonary artery
Left pulmonary veins
Auricle of left atrium
Circumflex artery
Left coronary artery (in coronary sulcus)
Left ventricle
Anterior interventricular artery (in anterior interventricular sulcus)
Apex

CIRCULATORY PROBLEMS

There are many disorders associated with circulatory problems, which exist when oxygenated blood cannot make the complete circuit of the body without restriction. There are many reasons why blood flow around the body may be inhibited. Clots may form in the larger veins in the leg or pelvic area, travel to the lung, and become trapped in a pulmonary artery. This results in diminished blood flow and less oxygen getting pumped to the rest of the body. *Pulmonary embolism,* as this condition is called, is difficult to detect, but is usually accompanied by a sudden shortness of breath and can be life-threatening.

When plaque or fatty deposits form along the walls of the arteries, it causes them to harden and constrict. *Hypertension*, or high blood pressure, results because the blood exerts greater force against the walls of the narrowed and/or rigid blood vessels. Hypertension can lead to stroke, angina pectoris (chest pain), kidney damage, and heart attack.

A circulatory disease that is brought on by chronic inflammation of the blood vessels in the extremities is *thromboangiitis obliterans (Buerger's disease).* This disease is most prevalent among people who smoke. It usually affects the foot or lower leg, but it can occur in the hand, arm, or thigh as well. Early signs of Buerger's disease are a tingling sensation (commonly referred to as "pins and needles") and a burning sensation in the fingers and toes. It can lead to ulceration and gangrene; in severe cases, amputation may be required.

Another serious circulatory condition is *Raynaud's disease,* which is characterized by constriction and spasm of the blood vessels in the extremities, such as in the fingers, toes, and tip of the nose. Cold, stress, smoking, and other factors may cause fingers and toes to become numb; extremities may appear colorless or bluish due to lack of circulation and arterial spasm. This disorder most commonly affects women between fifteen and fifty, and although it is extremely rare, it can lead to dry gangrene if tissue dies because of a lack of oxygen. *Raynaud's phenomenon* is a condition with the same symptoms as Raynaud's disease, but it is brought on by another condition, such as surgery, injury, or frostbite. Raynaud's may be provoked or aggravated by some heart medications and drugs taken for migraine, lupus, and rheumatoid arthritis.

Marfan's syndrome, a very rare condition, can also lead to serious circulatory problems. This syndrome is characterized by defects of the connective tissue in areas such as the skeletal system, eyes, and blood vessels, as well as such anatomical anomalies as unusually long toes and/or fingers, a high palate, an enlarged aorta, and/or taller than average height. This condition is usually hereditary.

Poor circulation can also result from *varicose veins,* which develop because of a loss of elasticity in the walls of the veins.

NUTRIENTS

SUPPLEMENT	SUGGESTED DOSAGE	COMMENTS
ESSENTIAL		
L-Carnitine	500 mg twice daily.	Helps to strengthen the heart Muscle and to promote Circulation by transporting long Fatty acid chains.
VERY IMPORTANT		
Chlorophyll (Kyo-Green from Wakunaga and Wheatgrass are Good sources)	As directed on label.	Enhances circulation and helps build healthy cells. Use liquid or tablet form. Also prepare fresh "green drinks" from green leafy vegetables.
Coenzyme Q10 Plus	100 mg daily.	Improves tissue oxygenation.
Coenzyme A From Coenzyme A Technologies	As directed on label.	Removes toxic substances from the body.
Lecithin granules Or Capsules	1 tblsp 3 times daily, before meals. 2,400 mg 3 times daily, Before meals.	Emulsifies (breaks up) fats.
Liquid Kyolic With B1 and B12 From Wakunaga	As directed on label.	Helps to build red blood cells and lower blood pressure.
Multienzyme Complex	As directed on label. Take with meals.	To aid digestion and circulation And enhance oxygen use in all Body tissues.
Vitamin B complex	50-100 mg of each major B vitamin 3 times daily (amounts of individual Vitamins in a complex Will vary)	Needed for metabolism of fat and cholesterol. Consider injections (under a doctor's supervision). If injections are not available, use a sublingual form.
Plus extra Vitamin B1 (thiamine) And	50 mg daily.	Enhances circulation and brain function.
Vitamin B6 (pyridoxine)	50 mg daily.	A natural diuretic that protects the heart.

And		
Vitamin B12	1,000-2,000 mcg daily.	Prevents anemia and acts as a natural energy booster.
And		
Folic acid	300 mcg daily.	Needed for the formation of oxygen-carrying red blood cells
And		
Para-aminobenzoic Acid (PABA)	25 mcg daily.	Assists in the formation of red blood cells.
Vitamin C With Bioflavonoids	5,000-10,000 mg daily. in divided doses.	Helps prevents blood clotting.
IMPORTANT Calcium	1,500-2,000 mg daily, In divided doses, after Meals and at bedtime.	Essential in normal blood viscosity.
And Magnesium	750-1,000 mg daily, In divided doses, after meals and at bedtime.	Strengthens the heartbeat. Calcium and magnesium Work together.
And Vitamin D3	400 IU daily.	Important for utilization of Calcium.
Dimethylglycine (DMG) (Aangamilk DMG from FoodScience of Vermont)	50 mg twice daily.	Enhances tissues oxygenation.
Multivitamin and Mineral complex	As directed on label.	To provide a balance of nutrients basic to good Circulatory function.
Vinpocetine	As directed on label.	A derivative of vincimine, (an Extract of periwinkle) that Helps with cerebral circulatory Disorders.
Vitamin A With Mixed caroteniods	25,000 IU daily. If you are pregnant, do not exceed 10,000 IU daily.	Aids in storage of fat and acts as an antioxidant. Use emulsion Form for easier assimilation and Greater safety at high doses.
And Vitamin E	Start with 200 IU daily	Inhibits the formation of free Radicals. Use d-alpha-tocopherol Form; use emulsion form for Best absorption.

Choline And Inositol Plus	100 mg each 3 times daily, with meals.	Helps to remove fat deposits And improve circulation. Helps to lower cholesterol.
Vitamin B3 (niacin)	50 mg 3 times daily. Do not exceed a total Of 300 mg daily from All supplements.	Helps lower cholesterol. *Caution:* do not take niacin if you have a liver disorder, Gout, or high blood pressure.
L-cysteine And L-methionine	500 mg each daily, on An empty stomach. Take with juice or water. Do not take with milk. Take With 50 mg vitamin B6 And 100 mg vitamin C For better absorption.	Protects and preserves cells by detoxifying harmful toxins. Prevents accumulation of fat both in the liver and in the arteries, where it may obstruct Blood low.
Proteolytic enzymes	As directed on label. Take between meals.	To combat leaky gut syndrome.
Pycnogenol Or Grape seed extract	As directed on label. As directed on label.	Neutralize free radicals, enhance the action of vitamin C, and strengthen connective tissue, Including that of the cardio- Vascular system.
Selenium	200 mcg daily. If you Are pregnant, do not Exceed 40 mcg daily.	Deficiency has been linked to heart disorders.
Shiitake extract Or Reishi extract	As directed on label. As directed on label.	Helps to prevent high blood pressure and heart disease; lowers cholesterol levels.
Zinc plus Copper	50 mg daily. Do not Exceed a total of 100 mg daily from all supplements. 3 mg daily.	Needed for immune function. Use zinc chelate form. Needed to balance with zinc.

HERBS

- The following herbs support the heart and circulatory system: black cohosh, butcher's broom, cayenne (capsicum), chickweed, gentian root, ginkgo biloba, goldenseal, hawthorn berries, horseradish, horsetail, hyssop, licorice root, pleurisy root, rose hips, and wormwood. Cayenne increases the pulse rate, while black cohosh slows it. Ginkgo is being used for circulatory disorders in many clinics.

    Caution: Do not use black cohosh if you are pregnant or have any type of chronic disease. Do not use licorice on a daily basis for more than 7 days in a row, and avoid it completely if you have high blood pressure. Do not use wormwood during pregnancy. It is not recommended for long-term use, as it is habit-forming.

- Sanhelio's Circu Caps from Health From The Sun is an herbal combination formula beneficial for circulatory disorders.

RECOMMENDATIONS

- Make sure your diet is high in fiber. Oat bran can help lower cholesterol levels.

- Include the following in your diet: bananas, brown rice, endive, garlic, lima beans, onions, pears, peas, and spinach.

- Drink steam-distilled water only.

- Eliminate animal protein and fatty foods (such as red meat), sugar, and white flour from your diet. Do not use stimulants such as coffee, colas, or tobacco, or eat foods with a lot of spices.

- Get regular exercise to help blood flow and to keep the arteries soft and unclogged.

    Caution: If you are over thirty-five and/or have been sedentary for some time, consult your health care provider before beginning any type of any exercise program.

- Keep your weight down.

- To boost circulation, give yourself a dry massage over your entire body using a loofah sponge or natural bath brush. Always massage towards the heart, even when massaging your legs. Also dip a towel in cold water and rub it briskly over your body.

- If you have circulatory problems, do not take any preparations containing shark cartilage unless specifically directed to do so by your physician. Shark cartilage inhibits the formation of new blood vessels, the mechanism by which the body can increase circulatory capacity.

CONSIDERATIONS

- Blood-thinning drugs, such as warfarin (Coumadin), may be prescribed for people deemed to be in particular danger of developing blood clots, such as people who are bedridden or cancer patients. Studies show that, for those in peril of recurring clots, blood-thinning drugs should be taken for at least two years.

- Because sluggish circulation can have a variety of different causes, you should see your health care provider if it is persistent.

- Chelation therapy is helpful for improving circulation.

- The simple fact of being pregnant places great strain on the circulatory system. Blood volume increases by up to 50 percent by the time a woman is nine months pregnant, and although most woman with heart disease can safely have children, any such pregnancy should be closely monitored by both a cardiologist and an obstetrician.

Good Food Combinations

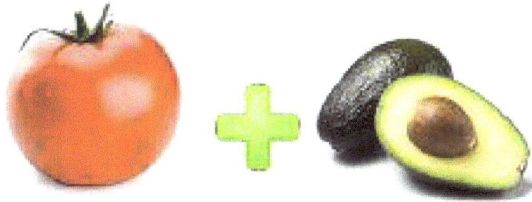

Tomatoes are rich in **lycopene**, a pigment-rich antioxidant known as a carotenoid, which reduces cancer risk and cardiovascular disease. Fats like avocado make carotenoids more bioavailable.

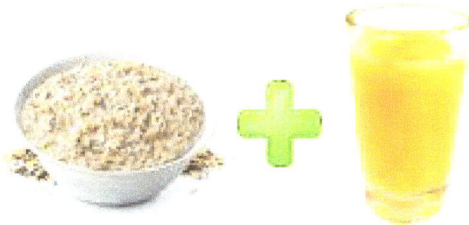

The organic compounds in both foods, called **phenols**, stabilize your LDL cholesterol (low-density lipoprotein, or so-called "bad" cholesterol) when consumed together.

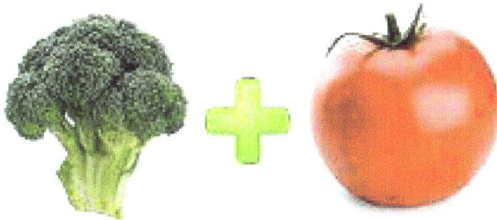

New research shows that this combo prevents prostate cancer, but no one is sure why.

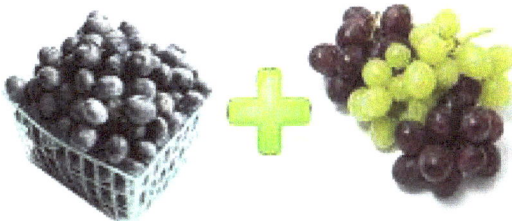

Studies have shown that the antioxidant effects of consuming a combination of fruits are more than additive but **synergistic**.

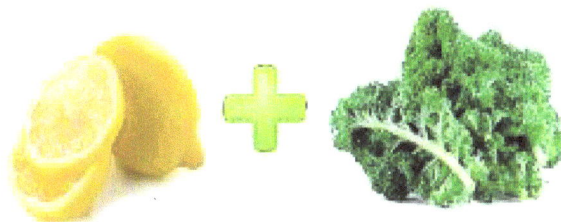

Vitamin C helps make plant-based iron more absorbable

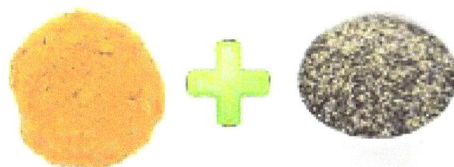

Adding black pepper to turmeric or turmeric-spiced food enhances curcumin's bioavailability by **1,000 times**

Emotional Intelligence Central

Strategies and Tips for Good Mental Health, I will give you the tools for lasting results.

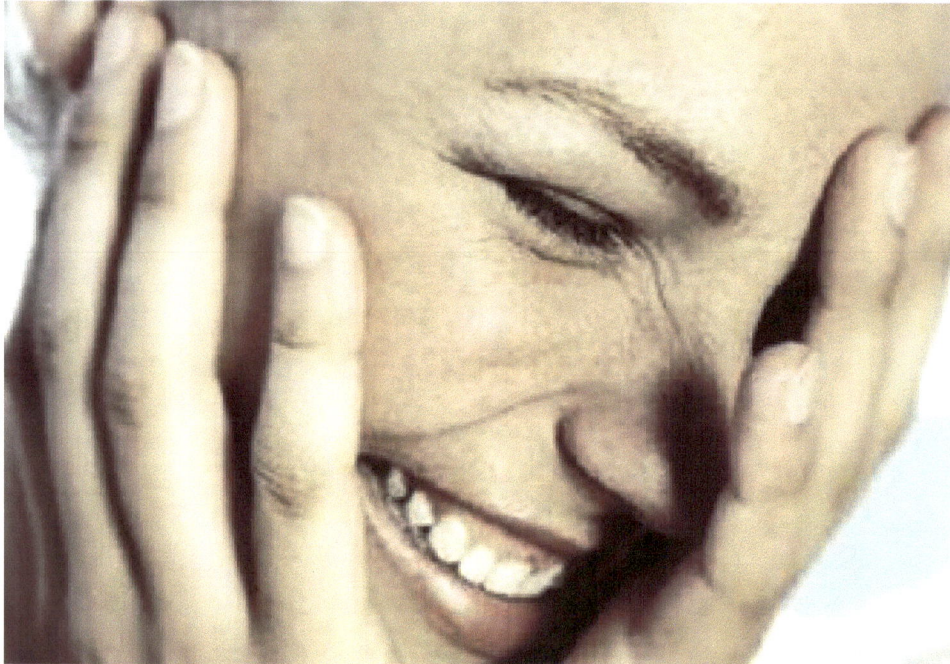

People who are emotionally healthy are in control of their emotions and their behavior. They are able to handle life's inevitable challenges, build strong relationships, and lead productive, fulfilling lives. When bad things happen, they're able to bounce back and move on.

Unfortunately, too many people take their mental and emotional health for granted – focusing on it only when they develop problems. But just as it requires effort to build or maintain physical health, so it is with mental and emotional health. The more time and energy you invest in your emotional health, the stronger it will be. The good news is that there are many things you can do to boost your mood, build resilience, and get more enjoyment out of life.

What is mental health or emotional health?

Mental or emotional health refers to your overall psychological well-being. It includes the way you feel about yourself, the quality of your relationships, and your ability to manage your feelings and deal with difficulties.

Good mental health isn't just the absence of mental health problems. Being mentally or emotionally healthy is much more than being free of depression, anxiety, or other psychological issues. Rather than the absence of mental illness, mental and emotional health refers to the presence of positive characteristics.

People who are mentally and emotionally healthy have:

- A sense of contentment.
- A zest for living and the ability to laugh and have fun.
- The ability to deal with stress and bounce back from adversity.
- A sense of meaning and purpose, in both their activities and their relationships.
- The flexibility to learn new things and adapt to change.
- A balance between work and play, rest and activity, etc.
- The ability to build and maintain fulfilling relationships.
- Self-confidence and high self-esteem.

These positive characteristics of mental and emotional health allow you to participate in life to the fullest extent possible through productive, meaningful activities and strong relationships. These positive characteristics also help you cope when faced with life's challenges and stresses.

The role of resilience in mental and emotional health

Being emotionally and mentally healthy doesn't mean never going through bad times or experiencing emotional problems. We all go through disappointments, loss, and change. And while these are normal parts of life, they can still cause sadness, anxiety, and stress.

The difference is that people with good emotional health have an ability to bounce back from adversity, trauma, and stress. This ability is called *resilience*. People who are emotionally and mentally healthy have the tools for coping with difficult situations and maintaining a positive outlook. They remain focused, flexible, and creative in bad times as well as good.

One of the key factors in resilience is the ability to balance your emotions. The capacity to recognize your emotions and express them appropriately helps you avoid getting stuck in depression, anxiety, or other negative mood states. Another key factor is having a strong support network. Having trusted people you can turn to for encouragement and support will boost your resilience in tough times.

Building your resilience

Resilience involves maintaining flexibility and balance in your life as you deal with stressful circumstances and traumatic events. This happens in several ways, including:

- Letting yourself experience strong emotions, and also realizing when you may need to avoid experiencing them at times in order to continue functioning
- Stepping forward and taking action to deal with your problems and meet the demands of daily living, and also stepping back to rest and reenergize yourself
- Spending time with loved ones to gain support and encouragement, and also nurturing yourself
- Relying on others, and also relying on yourself. (*Source: American Psychological Association*)

Physical health is connected to mental and emotional health

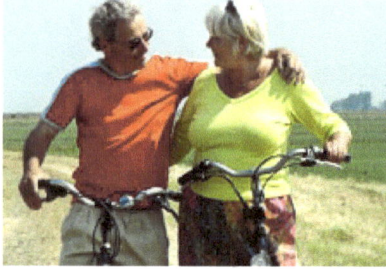

Taking care of your body is a powerful first step towards mental and emotional health. The mind and the body are linked. When you improve your physical health, you'll automatically experience greater mental and emotional well-being. For example, exercise not only strengthens our heart and lungs, but also releases endorphins, powerful chemicals that energize us and lift our mood.

The activities you engage in and the daily choices you make affect the way you feel physically and emotionally.

- **Get enough rest.** To have good mental and emotional health, it's important to take care of your body. That includes getting enough sleep. Most people need seven to eight hours of sleep each night in order to function optimally.
- **Learn about good nutrition and practice it**. The subject of nutrition is complicated and not always easy to put into practice. But the more you learn about what you eat and how it affects your energy and mood, the better you can feel.
- **Exercise to relieve stress and lift your mood**. Exercise is a powerful antidote to stress, anxiety, and depression. Look for small ways to add activity to your day, like taking the stairs instead of the elevator or going on a short walk. To get the most mental health benefits, aim for 30 minutes or more of exercise per day.
- **Get a dose of sunlight every day**. Sunlight lifts your mood, so try to get at least 10 to 15 minutes of sun per day. This can be done while exercising, gardening, or socializing.
- **Limit alcohol and avoid cigarettes and other drugs.**

Improve mental and emotional health by taking care of yourself

In order to maintain and strengthen your mental and emotional health, it's important to pay attention to your own needs and feelings. Don't let stress and negative emotions build up. Try to maintain a balance between your daily responsibilities and the things you enjoy. If you take care of yourself, you'll be better prepared to deal with challenges if and when they arise.

Tips and strategies for taking care of yourself:

- **Appeal to your senses**. Stay calm and energized by appealing to the five senses: sight, sound, touch, smell, and taste. Listen to music that lifts your mood, place flowers where you will see and smell them, massage your hands and feet, or sip a warm drink.
- **Engage in meaningful, creative work**. Do things that challenge your creativity and make you feel productive, whether or not you get paid for it – things like gardening, drawing, writing, playing an instrument, or building something in your workshop.
- **Get a pet**. Yes, pets are a responsibility, but caring for one makes you feel needed and loved. There is no love quite as unconditional as the love a pet can give. Animals can also get you out of the house for exercise and expose you to new people and places.
- **Make leisure time a priority**. Do things for no other reason than that it feels good to do them. Go to a funny movie, take a walk on the beach, listen to music, read a good book, or talk to a friend. Doing things just because they are fun is no indulgence. Play is an emotional and mental health necessity.
- **Make time for contemplation and appreciation.** Think about the things you're grateful for. Mediate, pray, enjoy the sunset, or simply take a moment to pay attention to what is good, positive, and beautiful as you go about your day.

Everyone is different; not all things will be equally beneficial to all people. Some people feel better relaxing and slowing down while others need more activity and more excitement or stimulation to feel better. The important thing is to find activities that you enjoy and that give you a boost.

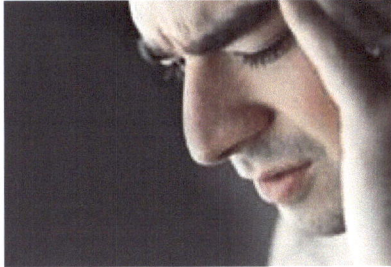

Limit unhealthy mental habits like worrying

Try to avoid becoming absorbed by repetitive mental habits – negative thoughts about yourself and the world that suck up time, drain your energy, and trigger feelings of anxiety, fear, and depression.

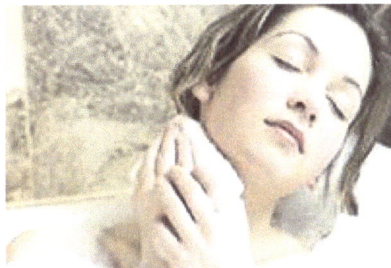

Manage your stress levels

Stress takes a heavy toll on mental and emotional health, so it's important to keep it under control. While not all stressors can be avoided, stress management strategies can help you brings things back into balance.

For tips on how to reduce, prevent, and cope with stress.

Supportive relationships: The foundation of emotional health

No matter how much time you devote to improving your mental and emotional health, you will still need the company of others to feel and be your best. Humans are social creatures with emotional needs for relationships and positive connections to others.. We're not meant to survive, let alone thrive, in isolation. Our social brains crave companionship—even when experience has made us shy and distrustful of others.

Tips and strategies for connecting to others:

- **Get out from behind your TV or computer screen.** Screens have their place but they will never have the same effect as an expression of interest or a reassuring touch. Communication is a largely nonverbal experience that requires you to be in direct contact with other people, so don't neglect your real-world relationships in favor of virtual interaction.
- **Spend time daily, face-to-face, with people you like**. Make spending time with people you enjoy a priority. Choose friends, neighbors, colleagues, and family members who are upbeat, positive, and interested in you. Take time to inquire about people you meet during the day that you like.
- **Volunteer**. Doing something that helps others has a beneficial effect on how you feel about yourself. The meaning and purpose you find in helping others will enrich and expand your life. There is no limit

to the individual and group volunteer opportunities you can explore. Schools, churches, nonprofits, and charitable organization of all sorts depend on volunteers for their survival.

- **Be a joiner.** Join networking, social action, conservation, and special interest groups that meet on a regular basis. These groups offer wonderful opportunities for finding people with common interests – people you like being with who are potential friends.

Building Great Relationships

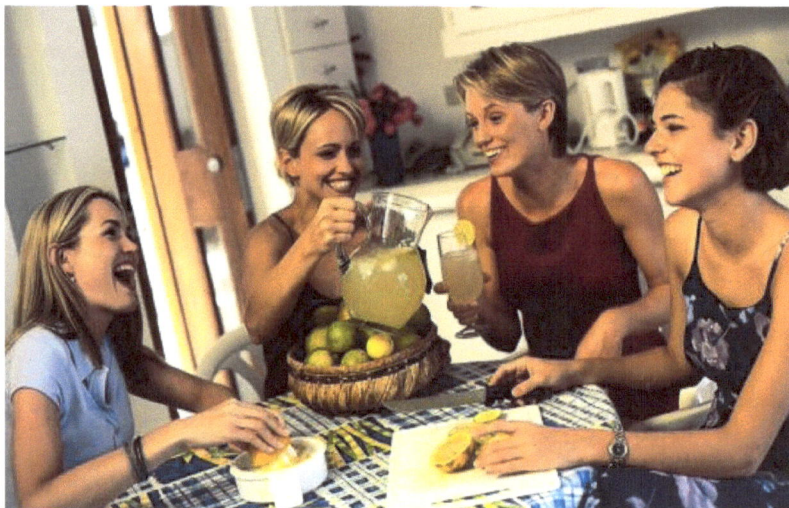

If you find it difficult to connect to others or to maintain fulfilling, long-term relationships, you may benefit from raising your emotional intelligence. Emotional intelligence allows us to communicate clearly, "read" other people, and resolve conflicts.

Risk factors for mental and emotional problems

Your mental and emotional health has been and will continue to be shaped by your experiences. Early childhood experiences are especially significant. Genetic and biological factors can also play a role, but these too can be changed by experience.

Risk factors that can compromise mental and emotional health:

- **Poor connection or attachment to your primary caretaker early in life.** Feeling lonely, isolated, unsafe, confused, or abused as an infant or young child.
- **Traumas or serious losses, especially early in life.** Death of a parent or other traumatic experiences such as war or hospitalization.
- **Learned helplessness.** Negative experiences that lead to a belief that you're helpless and that you have little control over the situations in your life.
- **Illness,** especially when it's chronic, disabling, or isolates you from others.
- **Side effects of medications**, especially in older people who may be taking a variety of medications.
- **Substance abuse**. Alcohol and drug abuse can both cause mental health problems and make preexisting mental or emotional problems worse.

Whatever internal or external factors have shaped your mental and emotional health, it's never too late to make changes that will improve your psychological well-being. Risk factors can be counteracted with protective factors, like strong relationships, a healthy lifestyle, and coping strategies for managing stress and negative emotions.

When to seek professional help for emotional problems

If you've made consistent efforts to improve your mental and emotional health and you still don't feel good – then it's time to seek professional help. Because we are so socially attuned, input from a knowledgeable, caring professional can motivate us to do things for ourselves that we were not able to do on our own.

The question of when to seek professional help can be answered by looking over the following list of red flags.

Red flag feelings and behaviors that require immediate attention

- Inability to sleep.
- Feeling down, hopeless, or helpless most of the time.
- Concentration problems that are interfering with your work or home life.
- Using smoking, overeating, drugs, or alcohol to cope with difficult emotions.
- Negative or self-destructive thoughts or fears that you can't control.
- Thoughts of death or suicide.

If you identify with any of these red flag symptoms, make an appointment with a mental health professional – and the sooner, the better. It's much easier to overcome a mental or emotional problem if you deal with it while it's small, rather than waiting until it's a major, entrenched problem.

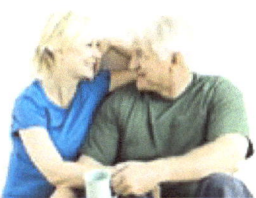 Emotional intelligence can help you strengthen your relationships, succeed at work, and overcome life's challenges.

Parsley is more than a garnish… Years pass by and our kidneys are filtering the blood by removing salt, poison and any unwanted entering our body. With time, the salt accumulates and this needs to undergo cleaning treatments and how are we going to overcome this? It is very easy, first take a bunch of parsley (MALLI Leaves)and wash it clean then cut it in small pieces and put it in a pot and pour clean water and boil it for ten minutes and let it cool down and then filter it and pour in a clean bottle and keep it inside refrigerator to cool. Drink one glass daily and you will notice all salt and other accumulated poison coming out of your kidney by urination also you will be able to notice the difference which you never felt before. Parsley is known as best cleaning treatment for kidneys and it is natural!

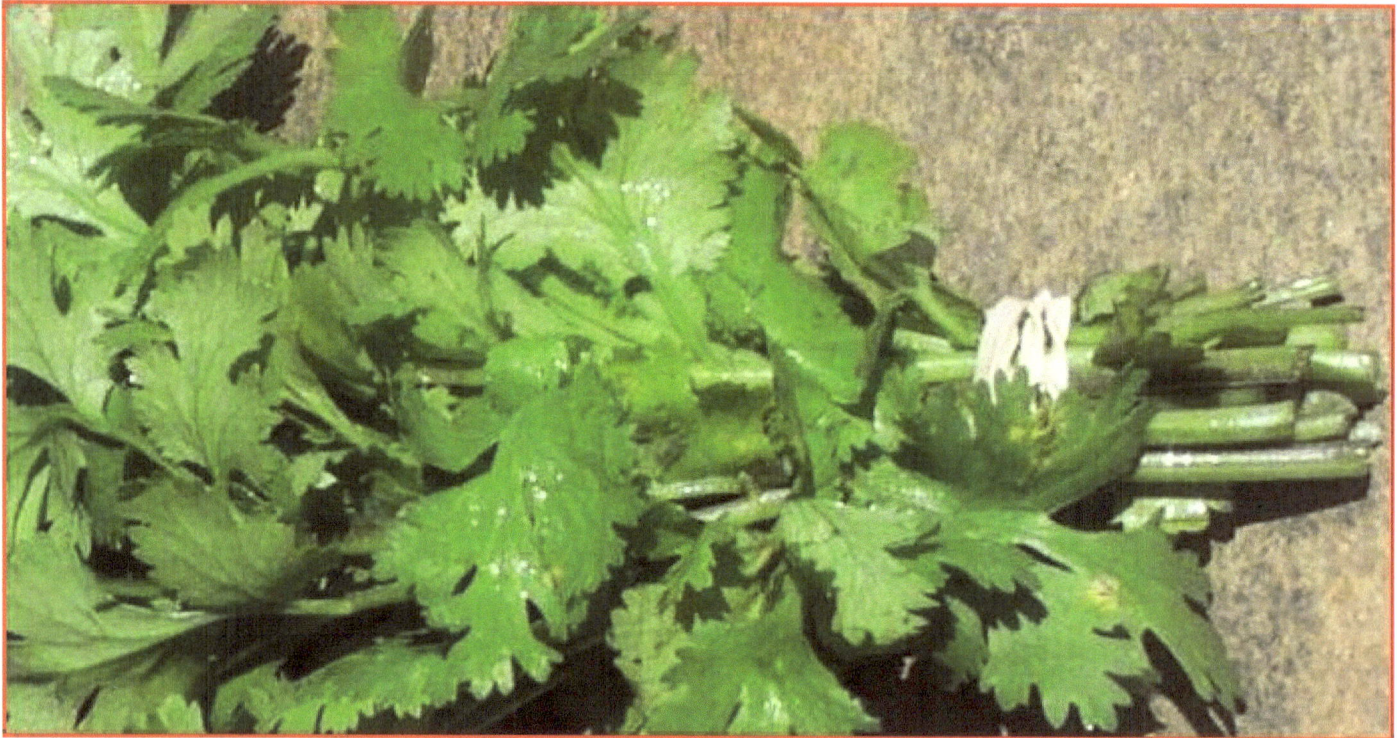

This is how your day of beverages should look for a healthy tomorrow...

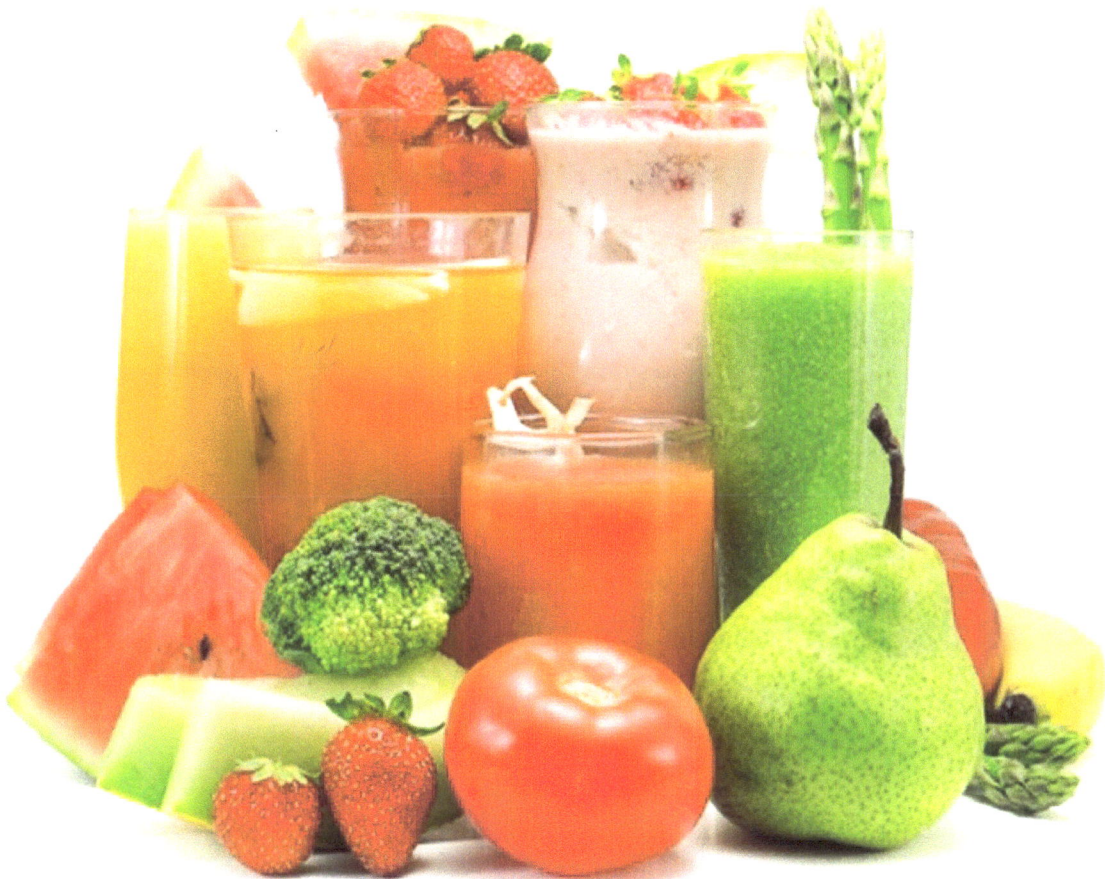

ULCERATIVE COLITIS

Ulcerative colitis is a chronic disorder in which the mucous membranes lining the colon become inflamed and develop ulcers, causing bloody diarrhea, pain, gas, bloating, and at times hard stools. The colon muscles then have to work harder to move these hardened stools through the colon. This can cause the mucous lining of the colon wall to bulge out into small pouchlike projections called diverticula. This usually occurs in the lower left section of the large intestine called the *sigmoid* ("S-shaped") colon, although it can occur in any part of the colon. *Enteritis* and *iletis* are types of inflammation of the small intestine often associated with colitis.

Ulcerative colitis can range from relatively mild to severe. Common complications are diarrhea, and bleeding, often causing the loss of vital nutrients and fluids. A rarer complication is toxic megacolon, in which the intestinal wall weakens and balloons out, threatening to rupture. The cause or causes of colitis are unknown, but possible contributing factors include poor eating habits, stress, and food allergies. Colitis can also be caused by infectious agents such as bacteria. This type of colitis is often associated with the use of antibiotics, which alter the normal bowel flora and permit microorganisms that are normally held in check to proliferate. The symptoms can range from simple diarrhea to the severe type of symptoms associated with ulcerative colitis.

Unless otherwise specified, the dosages recommended here are for adults. For children between the ages of twelve and seventeen, reduce the dose to three-quarters of the recommended amount. For a child between six and twelve, use one-half of the recommended dose, and for a child under the age of six, use one-quarter of the recommended amount.

SUPPLEMENT	SUGGESTED DOSAGE	COMMENTS
ESSENTIAL		
Iron	As directed by physician.	Usually depleted in people with Chronic inflammatory bowel Disease. *Note:* Do not take supplemental Iron unless anemia has been diagnosed .
Proteolytic enzymes	As directed on label. Take between meals.	Vital for proper digestion of Proteins and helps to control inflammation.
Plus		
Multienzyme complex	As directed on label. Take after meals.	Anti-inflammatory enzymes. Use a formula that is high
With		in pancreatin and low in
Pancreatin		Hydrochloric acid (HCL).
Vitamin B complex	As directed on label.	Essential for the breakdown of Fats, protein, and carbohydrates And for the proper digestion.
Plus extra		Use a hypoallergenic formula.
Vitamin B6	50 mg 2 times daily.	
And		
Vitamin B12	1,000 mcg twice daily.	A sublingual form is best.
And		
Folic acid	400 mcg twice daily.	Often depleted in people with This disorder. May protect Against colon cancer.

VERY IMPORTANT

Acidophilus (Kyo-Dophilus From Wakunaga Is a good source) Or Bio-Bifidus from American Biologics	As directed on label twice daily, on an empty stomach.	To normalize the intestinal bacteria. Very important if You are taking antibiotics. Use a nondairy formula.
Aerobic Bulk Cleanse From Aerobic Life Industries or Psyllium husks	1 tbsp in water or juice on an empty stomach in the morning. Drink it down quickly, before it thickens. Take separately from other Supplements and medications. As directed on label.	To keep the colon walls clean of toxic wastes.
Free-form amino Acid complex	As directed on label twice daily, on an Empty stomach.	To supply needed protein for tissue healing.
L-Glutamine	500 mg twice daily, on An empty stomach. Take With water or juice. Do Not take with milk. Take With 50 mg vitamin B6 And 100 mg vitamin C For better absorption.	A major metabolic fuel for the intestinal cells; maintains the villi, the absorption surfaces on the intestines.

Vitamin A
  With
Mixed carotenoids
  Incuding
Natural-beta-carotene
  And
Vitamin E
	25,000 IU daily. If you
	pregnant, do not
	exceed 10,000 IU daily.
	
	Up to 800 IU daily.
		An antioxidant that protects
		the mucous membranes
		And aids in healing.
		
		An antioxidant that promotes
		healing.
		Deficiency has been associated
		With bowel cancer. Use
		d-alpha-tocopherol form .

Aerobic 07 from Aerobic Life Industries Or Dioxychlor from American Biologics	As directed on label twice daily. 10-20 drops sublingually 1-2 times daily.	Provides stabilized oxygen To the colon and destroys unwanted bacteria. An important antibacterial, Antifungal, and antiviral agent.
Colloidal silver	As directed on label.	A natural broad-spectrum Antiseptic that fights infection, Subdues inflammation, and Promotes healing. Can be taken By mouth or applied topically.
Essential fatty acids (flaxseed oil and Primrose oil are Good sources)	As directed on label.	Important in cell formation. Protects the lining of the colon.

Garlic (Kyolic From Wakunaga)	2 capsules 3 times daily, with meals.	A natural antibiotic that has a Healing effect on the colon.
Glucosamine sulfate Or N-Acetylglucosamine (N-A-G from Source Naturals)	As directed on label. As directed on label.	An important component in the protective mucous secretions of the digestive tract.
Multimineral complex With Calcium And Chromium And Magnesium And Zinc	As directed on label.	Malabsorption of these essential minerals is a problem with colitis. Calcium also is needed for the prevention of cancer which may occur due to constant irritation. Use a high-potency formula.
Raw thymus Glandular	500 mg twice daily.	Important in immune function.
VitaCarte from Phoenix BioLabs Or Shark cartilage	As directed on label. As directed on label.	Contains pure bovine cartilage, which can be effective in improving ulcerative colitis.
Vitamin C With Bioflavonoids	3,000-5,000 mg daily, in divided doses.	Needed for immune function and Healing of mucous membranes. Use a buffered form.

HERBS

- Aerobic Bulk Cleanse (ABC) from Aerobic Life Industries contains healing herbs that cleanse the colon. Take it mixed with half fruit or vegetable juice and half aloe vera juice, before meals.

  Note: Always take this product separately from other supplements and medications.

- Alfalfa, taken in capsule or liquid form, supplies vitamin K and chlorophyll, needed for healing. Take it as directed on the product label three times daily.

- Aloe vera aids in healing the colon, thereby easing pain. Drink ½ cup of aloe vera juice in the morning and again at bedtime.

- Boswellia,bromelain, buchu leaves, and turmeric (curcumin) reduce inflammation.

- Burdock root, milk thistle, and red clover aid in cleansing the blood. Milk thistle also improves liver function.

- Chamomile, dandelion, feverfew, papaya, red clover, slippery elm, and yarrow extract or tea are beneficial for colitis, as is pau d' arco tea.

  Caution: Do not use chamomile on an ongoing basis, and avoid it completely if you are allergic to ragweed. Do not use feverfew during pregnancy.

- Lobelia tea is good to drink. Also use it as an enema for inflammation of the colon; it gives quick relief.

  Caution: Do not take lobelia internally on an ongoing basis.

- Nettle and quercetin aid in inhibiting allergic reactions.

RECOMMENDATIONS

- Do not wear clothing that is tight around the waist.

- For acute pain, try drinking a large glass of water. This aids in flushing out particles caught in the crevices of the colon, relieving pain.

- During a flare-up, consume only soft foods until the pain has subsided. Put oat bran or steamed vegetables through a blender. Add 1 tablespoon of oat or rice bran daily to cereals and juice to add the bulk needed for cleansing the colon. Or add 1 tablespoon of Aerobic Bulk Cleanse to juice and drink it on an empty stomach upon arising.

- Eat plenty of dark green leafy vegetables. These are rich sources of vitamin K. Vitamin K deficiency has been linked to ulcerative colitis.

- Try eating junior baby foods for two weeks. Baby foods are easy to digest. Earth's Best baby foods are organic and are available in many health food stores and supermarkets. While on the baby food diet, take extra fiber such as glucomannan. Glucomannan should be taken one-half to one hour before meals with large glass of water.

  Note: Always take supplemental fiber separately from other supplements and medications.

- Do stretching exercises and take proteolytic enzymes to improve digestion.

- Use cleansing enemas made with 2 quarts of lukewarm water. This helps to rid the colon of undigested foods and relieve pain. Use wheatgrass juice as a retention enema. For severe gas and bloating, use an *L.bifidus* enema.

CONSIDERATIONS

- A food sensitivity test is advised for anyone who suffers from colitis. We have seen many people with colitis do well once they make changes to their diet and lifestyle.

- When magnesium is given intravenously with vitamin B6, it relaxes the muscles in the walls of the bowels and can control an attack of spastic colon.

- If serious complications arise and all other treatments have failed, surgery may be required.

- Vitamin K deficiency has been linked to ulcerative colitis. Sulfa drugs and mineral oil deplete vitamin K.

- Ulcerative colitis and Cron's disease are both classified as inflammatory bowel diseases. Irritable bowel syndrome (IBS), although capable of causing some similar symptoms, is a condition that involves no inflammation.

- The earliest signs of ulcerative colitis sometimes mimic the symptoms of arthritis-achiness and joint pain. These symptoms may or may not be accompanied by the abdominal discomfort typical of colitis. If you start experiencing arthritis-like symptoms, it may be beneficial to change your diet and see if improvement results.

- Anyone who has had ulcerative colitis for at least five years-even if it is mild or inactive for a long time-should undergo regular colonoscopy, since people with this disease run a much greater risk of developing colon cancer than the general population. A colonoscopy is an examination performed with a long, flexible instrument that allows a physician to see inside the length of the colon.

Pomegranate - The Anti-Cancer fruit.

* A pomegranate contains 3 times the levels of antioxidants found in Green Tea. In fact it contains more antioxidants than any other natural food source.

* Pomegranates are loaded with nutrition and are particularly abundant in vitamin C, potassium, & pantothenic acid (B5).

* A single pomegranate contains approx 40% of our recommended daily dose of vitamin C !

* High in fiber and FAT FREE.

* It is a rich source of vitamins A, E and folic acid.

* A pomegranate contains 3 times the levels of antioxidants found in Green Tea and red wine. In fact it contains more antioxidants than any other natural food source.

* Has powerful Anti-Carcinogenic properties "anti-cancer" especially Prostate Gland, Colon & Intestinal tissues- It is rich in anti-oxidant which have incredible free-radical scavenging effects that are just now being studied by scientists.

* Reduce bad LDL cholesterol levels, so keeping arteries from clotting and helping to prevent atherosclerosis, stroke and heart attacks.

* Good for your heart: The polyphenol anti-oxidants within Pomegranates are powerfully effective at preventing the oxidation of lipids and endothelial tissue which are the steps that produce atherosclerosis and heart disease.

* Stabilize blood pressure.

* Powerfully boost the Immune system, this makes pomegranate a powerful anti-infection and cancer cell destroying tool.

* Prevent infection.

* Reduce risk of developing Breast Cancer.

* Due to the high sugar content of fruit juices it is always advisable to either eat the entire fruit or drink just small quantities of the juice. The fruit itself contains a high content of fiber that slows down the release of the fruit sugars into the bloodstream. The rich array of anti-oxidants is also in its most pure form within the covering of a freshly ripened pomegranate. The juice does have many beneficial factors and due to pomegranates incredible anti-oxidant potency

SIMPLY SAID: Pomegranate is considered a SUPER FOOD because it contains high amounts of the antioxidants your body needs to stay healthy and strong.

Unusual Uses of Pomegranate

Can protect against osteoarthritis
High in vitamin C and potassium
Nausea and morning sickness
Loaded with antioxidants
Boost the immune system
Teeth and gum disorder
Dysentery and diarrhea
Anti-inflammatory
Intestinal worms
Ellagic acid
Anti aging
Stroke
Fever
Cancer
Arthritis
Loss of voice
Stomachache
Poor appetite

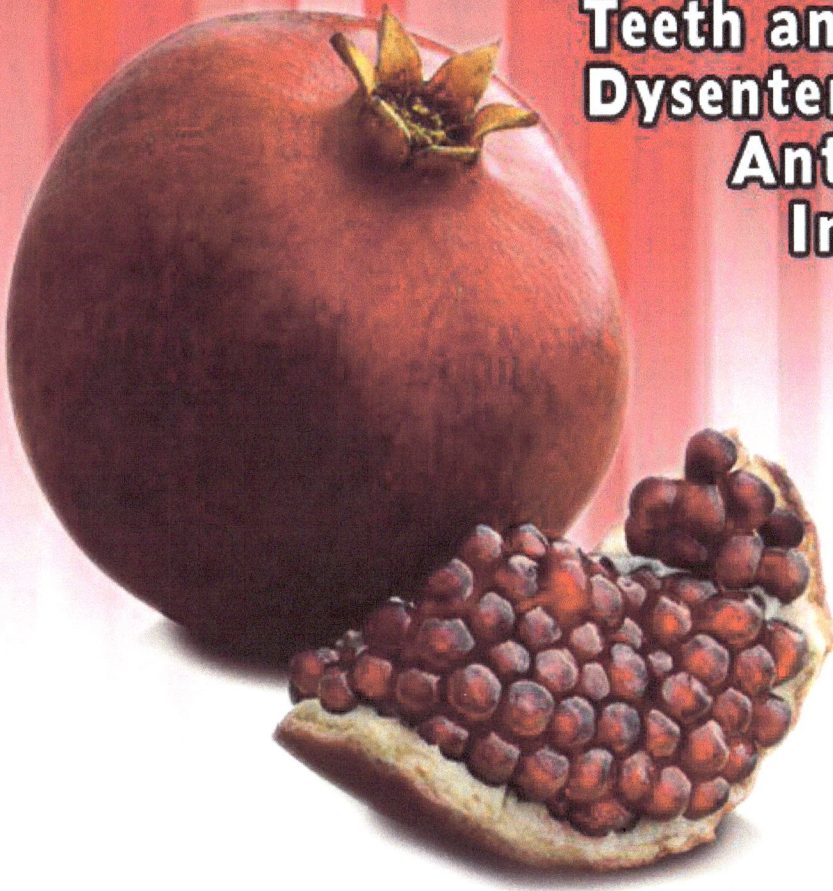

DIET FOR COLITIS

Ulcerative colitis can be an extremely painful and even temporarily disabling condition. Diet is probably the most significant factor in achieving and maintaining remission. Shari Lieberman, nutritionist and author, recommends the following dietary guidelines for people with colitis:

- Eat a low-carbohydrate, high-vegetable-protein diet. Include alfalfa or barley in diet. Baked or broiled fish, chicken, and turkey (without skin) are acceptable sources of protein.
- Eat lots of vegetables. If you cannot tolerate raw vegetables, steam them.
- Eat a high-fiber diet. Oat bran, brown rice, barley and other whole grains, lentils, and related products such as rice cakes are good. Be sure grains are well cooked.
- Keep fats and oils out of your diet, and stay away from high-fat milk and cheeses. Fats and oils exacerbate the diarrhea that comes from colitis.
- Include garlic in the diet for its healing and antibiotic properties.
- Eat cooked foods that broiled or baked, not fried or sautéed. Avoid sauces made with butter.
- Avoid carbonated soft drinks, spicy foods, and anything containing caffeine. These substances can irritate the colon. Also avoid red meat, sugar, and processed foods.
- Try soy-based cheese instead of dairy cheese; try soymilk or rice milk instead of cow's milk. If you eat dairy foods, use nonfat types. If you have a lactose intolerance, try lactose-free milk. Many lactose-intolerant people can tolerate low-fat yogurt.
- Drink plenty of liquids-at least 8-ounce glasses of water daily to make up for the fluid lost with diarrhea. Carrot and cabbage juices and "green drinks" are also good. Or add chlorophyll liquid to juices.
- Do not eat fruit on an empty stomach. Eat it between meals instead. Avoid acidic fruits such as oranges and grapefruit. Fruit juices should be diluted with water and taken during or after meals.

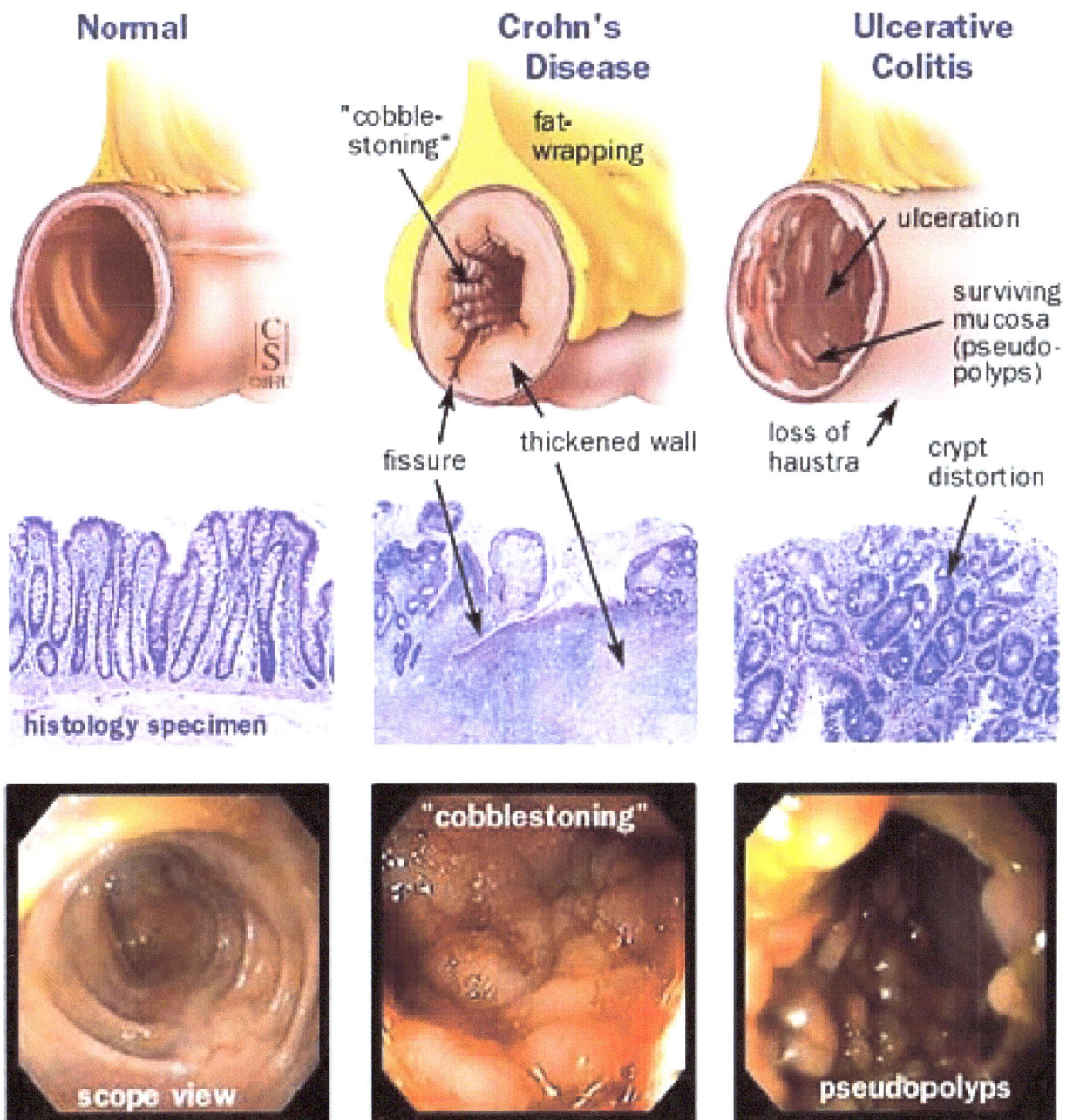

Normal

Crohn's Disease

"cobble-stoning"

fat-wrapping

fissure

thickened wall

Ulcerative Colitis

ulceration

surviving mucosa (pseudo-polyps)

loss of haustra

crypt distortion

histology specimen

scope view

"cobblestoning"

pseudopolyps

Figure 4. Gross (**top**), histological (**center**), and endoscopic (**bottom**) appearance of normal colon, Crohn's disease, and ulcerative colitis.

What Is Ehlers Danlos And What Are Some Home Treatments?

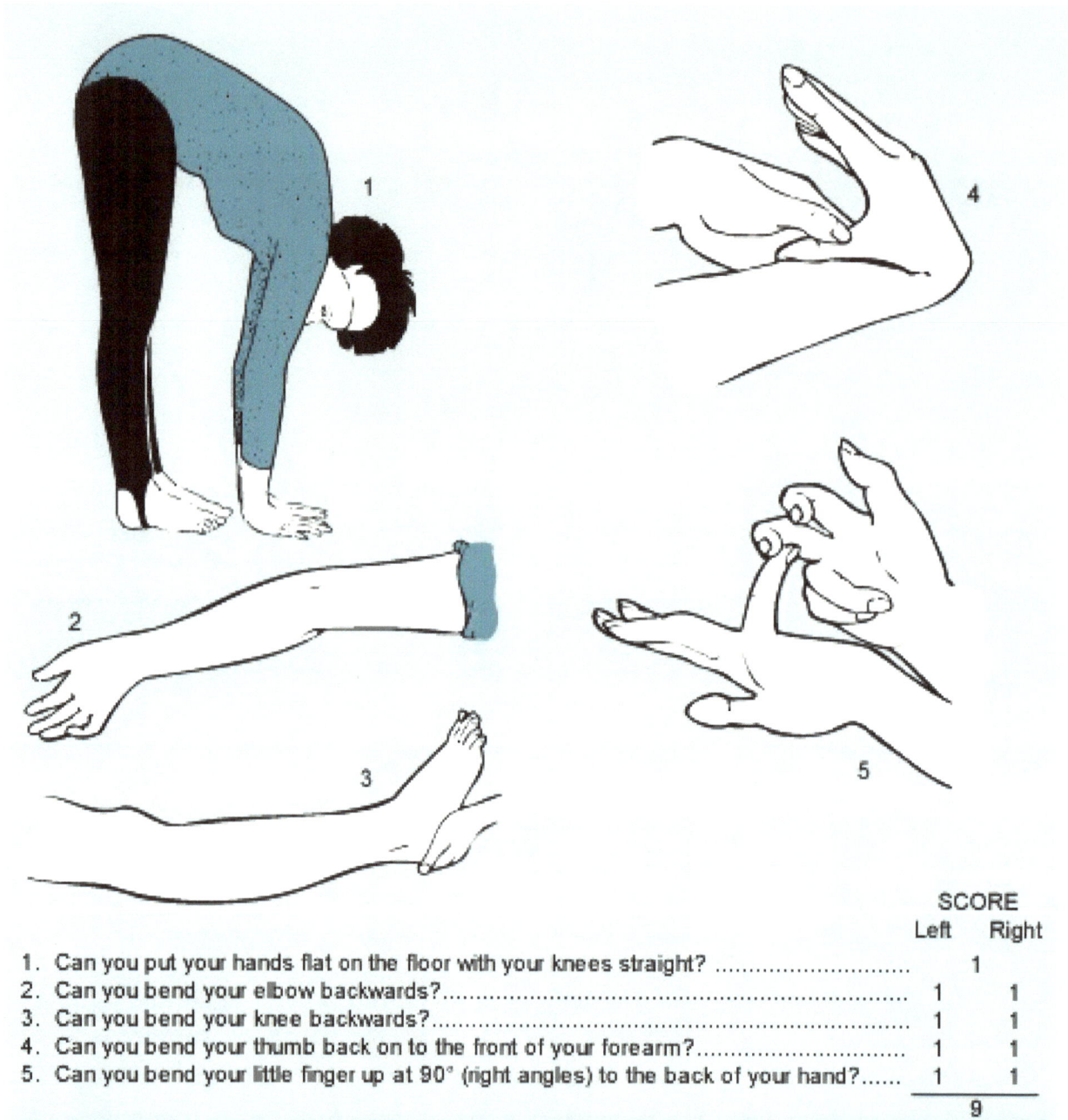

	SCORE	
	Left	Right
1. Can you put your hands flat on the floor with your knees straight?	1	
2. Can you bend your elbow backwards?...	1	1
3. Can you bend your knee backwards?...	1	1
4. Can you bend your thumb back on to the front of your forearm?...........................	1	1
5. Can you bend your little finger up at 90° (right angles) to the back of your hand?......	1	1
		9

Figure 1. Beighton's modification of the Carter and Wilkinson scoring system. Give youself 1 point for each of the manoeuvres you can do, up to a maximum of 9 points.

I was talking with a good friend the other day about a knee complaint her 12-year-old son was having after starting to run Cross Country for the first time. She said, "I need help." Her son was already very athletic, playing competitive travel baseball, as well as middle school baseball. He did plyometric training three times per week as well and did moderate (low weight) strength training in the gym. Basically, he was very fit and in shape. So he was asking, "Why me?" Why was he having pain?

Of course, pounding the pavement is hard on even the youngest, best, knees but it seemed like there must be something else at play as well. I didn't quite understand why a young athlete, in this top physical condition, would be having such discomfort so early into this new activity. I started digging into his medical history to see if I could find a way to help him.

Throughout the course of conversation, we found the key. My friend happened to mention that her son had been diagnosed with the mildest form of Ehlers-Danlos Syndrome (Class III) when he was 9. Ehlers-Danlos is made up of a group of syndromes of varying degrees but all generally classified as collagen-deficient connective tissue disorders at some level. The manifestations of Ehlers-Danlos are easy bruising, joint hypermobility (loose joints), skin that stretches easily (skin hyperelasticity or laxity), and weakness of tissues.

Even though my friend's son was very fit already, it was likely the manifestations of even his mild form of Ehler's-Danlos that were creating his knee pain symptoms! Once we had put this connection together, I immediately went to work on a plan using my knowledge of nutraceuticals and body dynamics. We came up with 3 simple things (plus one he was already doing and we just needed to reinforce it) to help overcome this knee pain.

Step 1:

Everyone with this disease - or any kind of joint/muscle pain - should be on baxyl which is far superior to glucosamine-condroitin-msm complex.

Step 2:

Everyone should also take a multi-vitamin/multi-mineral with Hyaluronic acid, vitamin E, Co-Q10,Conjugated Linoleic Acid (CLA), Omega fatty acid complex, and Flax Seed with Lignan. These all address the life support of your collagen with the added benefit of keeping your arterial walls pliable and reducing the chances of arterial sclerosis by assisting in the proper breakdown of plaque and cholesterol.

Step 3:

Use this "magic formula" recipe daily:

8 ounces of orange juice

8 ounces of Aloe Vera juice

1 scoop of Grapefruit pectin powder

2 tablespoon of lecithin

1 teaspoon of royal bee jelly

2 tablespoons of flax seed oil with lignin

1 tablespoon of bee pollen

1 tablespoon of "Trail Of Tears Beans" (a small jet black bean)

This recipe has a fruity/nutty flavor with the consistency of a smoothie. It has a multi-dimensional benefit in that it can be used as a meal replacement to help you lose body fat, build collagen, and emulsify the fat; thus, keep the arteries clean and clear. And it is good for your heart as well as your respiratory system!

Step 4:

Be thankful and realize that while you - or someone you love - is dealing with a very real physical disease, mental state is crucial in living with - and triumphing over - it. Luckily, my friend's son already had this part down. He understood the power of the mind and could tick off in a second, several reasons why he was actually thankful he had this disease. This was more than the power of positive thinking, he developed a full personal development plan and then executed it with commitment and dedication. I attribute that a lot to his mom who was consistently showing him how

the disease actually made him better at the things he did. For example, he was a starting first baseman on both middle school and competitive travel ball teams. The extreme flexibility caused by his Ehlers-Danlos meant he had the immense ability to stretch into complete splits - in every direction - to make the play. As a result, he had become known as the "best first baseman in his age group" in a tri-county area. The message behind all this is that when you - or your loved is faced with a "life-altering" illness or disease, remember that attitude is a huge part of dealing with it. Everything in life isperfect and is happening for a reason to serve you in your life in some way.

If you spend a little time/effort seeking how you (or they) are being served - in a positive manner - by this "seemingly-negative" situation, you will find you are able to triumph over it with less effort. Add a little good, old-fashioned, effort in the form of taking care of the physical manifestation of your body - right along with your spirit - and you can learn to say "Thank You God" for anything!

EDS Type	Major Diagnostic Criteria	Minor Diagnostic Criteria
Classical	Skin hyperextensibility, widened atrophic scars, joint hypermobility	• Positive family history
		• Physical findings include smooth velvety skin, mulluscoid pseudotumors, subcutaneous spheroids, complications of joint hypermobility (sprains, dislocations/subluxations), muscle hypotonia, delayed gross motor development, easy bruising, tissue extensibility, fragility, surgical complications
Hypermobility	Skin involvement (either smooth/velvety skin or hyperextensibility), generalized joint hypermobility	• Positive family history
		• Physical findings include recurring joint dislocations, chronic joint/limb pain
Vascular	Thin translucent skin, arterial/intestinal/uterine fragility or rupture, extensive bruising, characteristic facial appearance	• Positive family history, specifically sudden death of a close relative(s)
		• Physical findings include acrogeria, hypermobility of small joints, tendon and muscle rupture, clubfoot, early onset varicose veins, arteriovenous, carotid-cavernous sinus fistula, pneumothorax/pneumohemothorax, gingival recession
Kyphoscoliosis	Generalized joint laxity, severe muscle hypotonia at birth, scoliosis at birth, scleral fragility, rupture of the ocular globe	• Positive family history (e.g., affected siblings)
		• Physical findings include tissue fragility, atrophic scars, easy bruising, arterial rupture, marfanoid habitus (Marfan-like), microcornea, osteopenia on radiograph
Arthrochalasis	Severe generalized joint hypermobility with recurrent subluxations, congenital bilateral hip dislocation	• Physical findings include skin hyperextensibility, tissue fragility, atrophic scars, easy bruising, muscle hypotonia, kyphoscoliosis, osteopenia on radiograph
Dermatosparaxis	Severe skin fragility, sagging redundant skin	• Physical findings include soft, doughy skin, easy bruising, premature rupture of fetal membranes, large hernias (umbilical or inguinal)

How about this refreshing drink? It is a great feel good refresher and it is beautiful as it is delicious…

It's so easy-to-prepare and you only need fresh fruits, like peach, kiwi, lime and raspberries, and water. When you prepare it at home, you have always the option to skip the sugar.

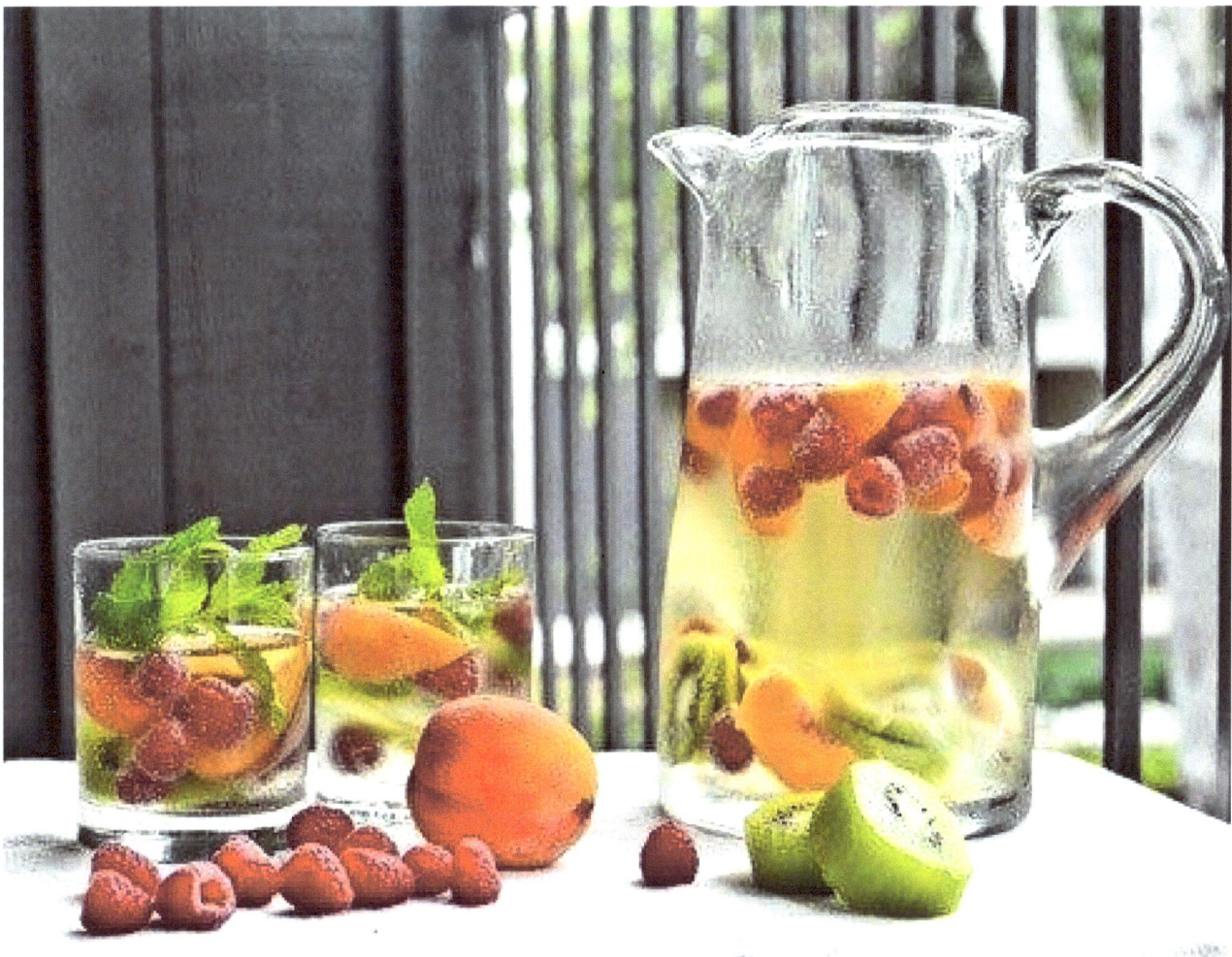

Step By Step
Turmeric Tea Recipe

1 cup of almond milk

1 teaspoon of turmeric root

1/2 teaspoon of black pepper

1/2 teaspoon of cumin

1/2 teaspoon of cinnamon

1/2 teaspoon of cardamon

1/2 teaspoon of coriander

1 teaspoon of honey or agave

Benefits Of Turmeric Tea

We all need a sweet treat from time to time and this is my go to drink. It smells heavenly and is a great drink either first thing in the morning or as a treat at the end of a long day.

1. It is a natural antiseptic and antibacterial agent, useful in disinfecting cuts and burns.
2. When combined with cauliflower, it has shown to prevent prostate cancer and stop the growth of existing prostate cancer.
3. Prevented breast cancer from spreading to the lungs in mice.
4. May prevent melanoma and cause existing melanoma cells to commit suicide.
5. Reduces the risk of childhood leukemia.
6. Is a natural liver detoxifier.
7. May prevent and slow the progression of Alzheimer's disease by removing amyloyd plaque buildup in the brain.
8. May prevent metastases from occurring in many different forms of cancer.
9. It is a potent natural anti-inflammatory that works as well as many anti-inflammatory drugs but without the side effects.
10. Has shown promise in slowing the progression of multiple sclerosis in mice.
11. Is a natural painkiller and cox-2 inhibitor.
12. May aid in fat metabolism and help in weight management.
13. Has long been used in Chinese medicine as a treatment for depression.
14. Because of its anti-inflammatory properties, it is a natural treatment for arthritis and rheumatoid arthritis.
15. Boosts the effects of chemo drug paclitaxel and reduces its side effects.
16. Promising studies are underway on the effects of turmeric on pancreatic cancer.
17. Studies are ongoing in the positive effects of turmeric on multiple myeloma.
18. Has been shown to stop the growth of new blood vessels in tumors.
19. Speeds up wound healing and assists in remodeling of damaged skin.
20. May help in the treatment of psoriasis and other inflammatory skin conditions.

According to Dr. Andrew Weil recent research on both turmeric and curcumin is very promising:

Curcumin seems to delay liver damage that can eventually lead to cirrhosis, according to preliminary experimental research at the Medical University Graz in Austria.

- Kansas State University research found that adding certain spices, including turmeric, can reduce the levels of heterocyclic amines — carcinogenic compounds that are formed when meats are barbecued, boiled or fried — by up to 40 percent

- Rodent studies at the University of Texas indicate that curcumin inhibits the growth of a skin cancer, melanoma and also slows the spread of breast cancer into the lungs.

- Researchers from the University of South Dakota have found that pretreatment with curcumin makes cancer cells more vulnerable to chemo and radiotherapy.

- Epidemiologists have hypothesized that the turmeric that is part of daily curries eaten in India may help explain the low rate of Alzheimer's disease in that country. Among people aged 70 to 79, the rate is less than one-quarter that of the United States.
- And at least one new study suggests **Curcumin's Value For Arthritis Treatment**. Since arthritis is so common and the results so interesting, it's worth a closer look.

Makes you want to make some tea doesn't it?

Ingredients:

1 cup Coconut Milk (or almond)

½ tspn Cinnamon

½ tspn Turmeric

1/8 tspn Nutmeg

Dash of Cayenne Pepper

Raw honey to taste

Instructions:

Put coconut milk, spices and honey in a saucepan heat up slowly on low heat. If you put it on high heat the coconut milk will get too thick. Pour and enjoy.

Source: www.healthy-holistic-living.com

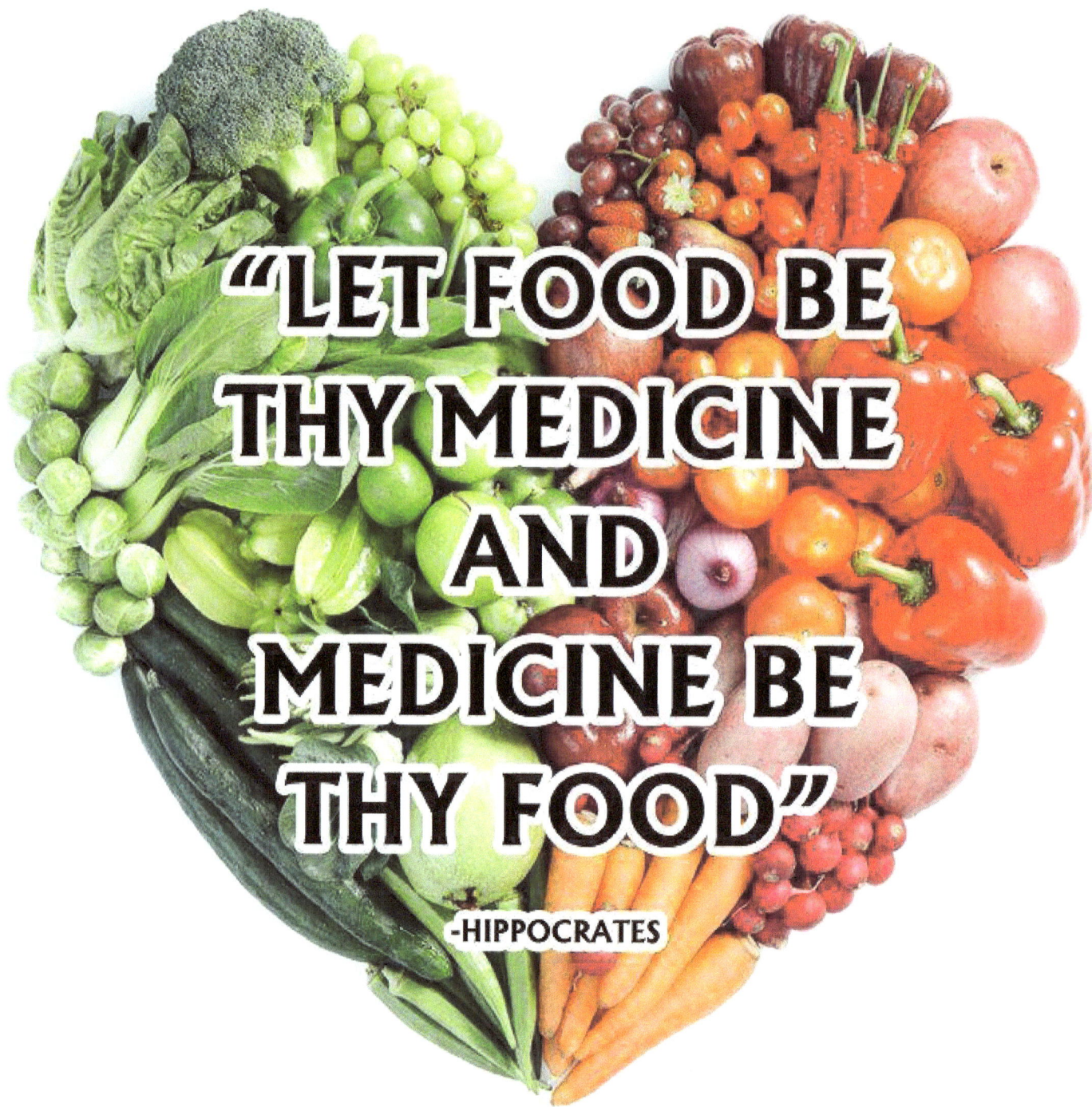

"LET FOOD BE THY MEDICINE AND MEDICINE BE THY FOOD"

-HIPPOCRATES

California Poppy is a medicinal herb and flower that is rich in vitamins A, C, and E as well as minerals such as calcium and magnesium. California poppy contains sedative properties that make it highly beneficial for relieving anxiety, stress, panic attacks, insomnia, hypertension, colic and bedwetting in children. It is also useful for behavioral disorders such as OCD, Bipolar disorder, Alzheimer's, ADD, and ADHD. California Poppy is good at sharpening cognitive skills such as memory and concentration which makes it a great herb for students and adults alike. California Poppy is known to be a phenomenal natural pain reliever and is a safe alternative to prescription medication. It contains analgesic and antispasmodic properties which is useful in providing relief from acute nerve and muscle related pain. California Poppy is also known to help reduce high fever, rapid pulse, and spasmodic coughs. California Poppy contains antimicrobial properties which makes it excellent for applying to cuts, wounds, and skin ailments. California poppy powder can be mixed with coconut oil as a natural treatment for the elimination of head lice. California Poppy tea is wonderful to drink before bed to help prepare the body for a full and restful night's sleep. Add 2 tsp of dried herb to 1 cup of boiling water and let steep for at least 10 minutes, sweeten with raw honey and/or lemon if desired. California Poppy can be found in tea, tincture, extract, capsule, and cream form online or at your local health food store.

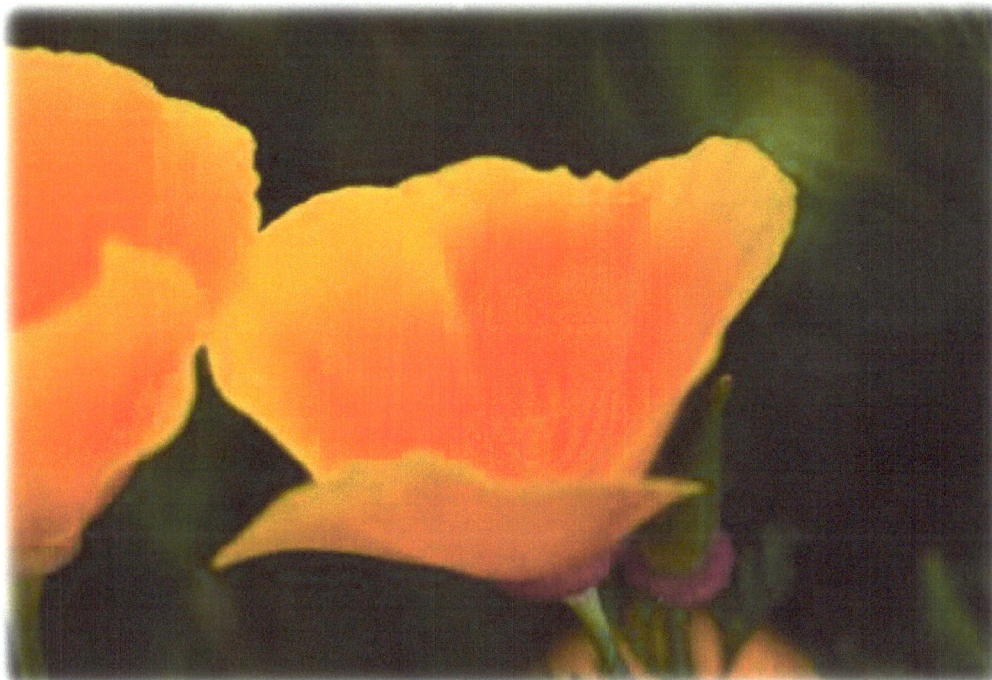

Green beans are a nutritious vegetable that are rich in vitamins, minerals, and phytonutrients such as vitamins A & C, calcium, iron, manganese, beta-carotene, and protein. Green beans provide signifiant cardiovascular benefits due to their omega-3 (alpha-linolenic acid) content. They also contain ant-inflammatory compounds which make them highly beneficial for individuals who suffer with auto-immune disorders such as fibromyalgia, arthritis, COPD, chronic fatigue syndrome, irritable bowl syndrome, chronic sinusitis, bursitis, Raynaud's syndrome and lupus. They are also known to help prevent type 2 diabetes. Green beans are an excellent source of dietary fiber and can aid the digestive tract by promoting regular peristaltic action and aid in the removal toxic, cancer-causing substances in the digestive tract. Green beans contain a wide variety of carotenoids such as lutein and neoxanthin and flavonoids such asquercetin and procyanidins which make them excellent for eye health and for preventing disease. Green beans can be snacked on raw, added to salads or soups, or steamed. Consider trying fresh green beans drizzled with olive oil, seasoned with your favorite spices, and roasted in the oven for 30 minutes for a healthy alternative to french fries. This crispy, savory snack is a great way to get kids and adults to love their vegetables. Fresh green beans are readily available at your local supermarket in the produce section. Also, keep a lookout at your local farmer's markets for heirloom varieties of green beans that contain the ultimate in nutritional and health benefits.

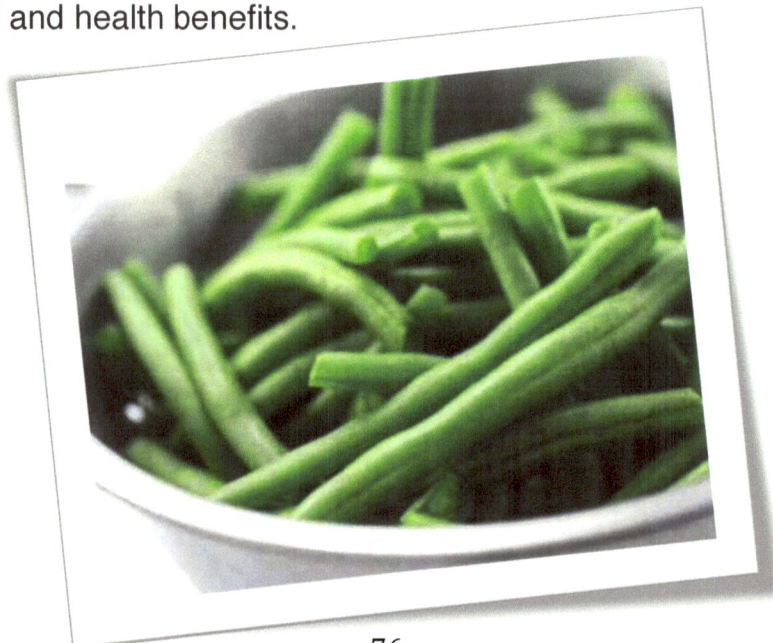

Cantaloupe is an amazing fruit that has over 19 vitamins and minerals that help to boost the immune system, detoxify the organs, and deeply hydrate and alkalinize the body. Since cantaloupe is a pre-digested food, meaning it does not require any digestion in the stomach and can pass straight through to the intestines for assimilation, it is best eaten on an empty stomach alone for breakfast. The high vitamin C content in cantaloupes is critical for immune system support and to fight bacterial and viral infections. Cantaloupe is also excellent for helping to relieve nerves and calm anxieties. It is known to keep the heartbeat normal and regulated while under stress as well as keep muscles relaxed and free from cramps and hypertension. The rich vitamin A and beta-carotene content in cantaloupe helps to lower the risk of cataracts and aids in maintaining healthy eyesight. Cantaloupe also aids the body in excreting excess sodium, which helps to reduce water tension and bloating. After purchasing a cantaloupe, let it sit on your counter until it emits a light floral scent and yields to gentle pressure. Cantaloupe is a sweet and delicious fruit that is a wonderful way to start your morning and nourish your body and soul.

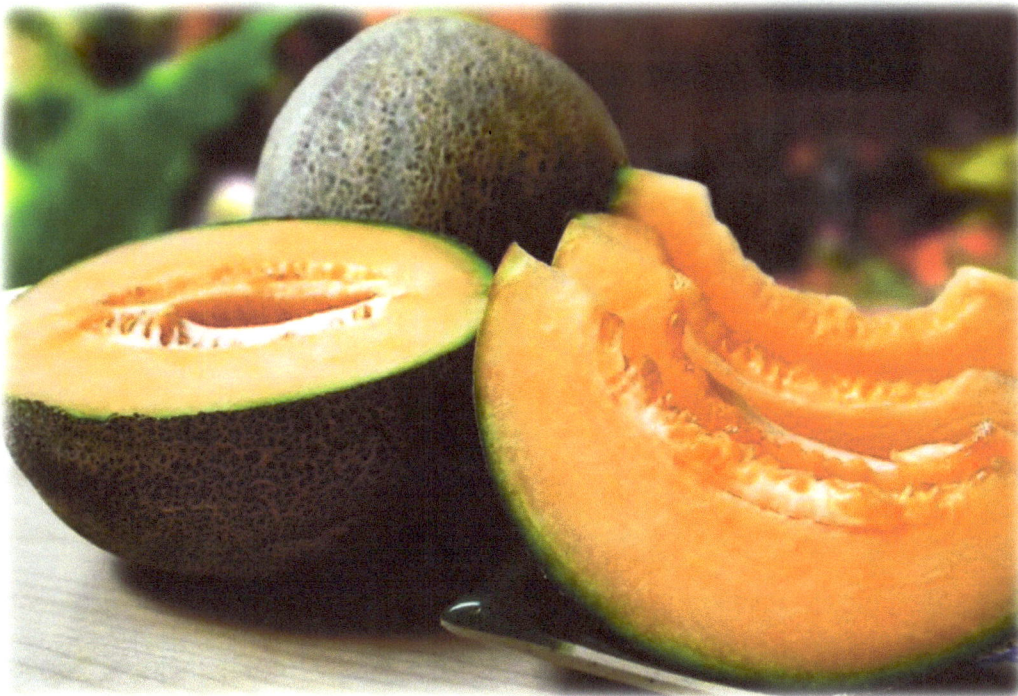

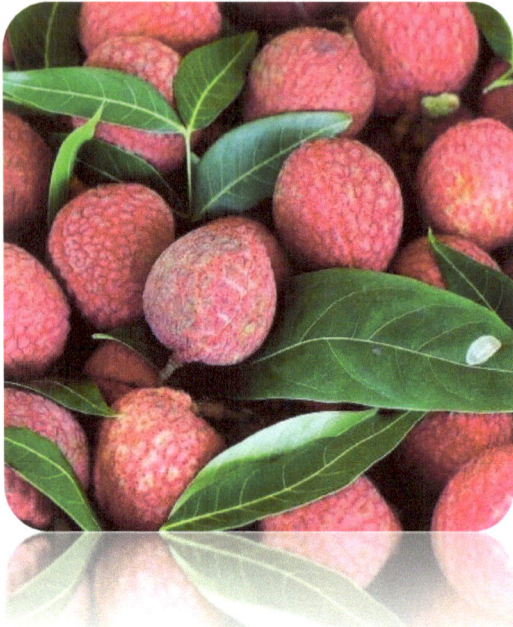

Lychee are a superfruit that are revered around the world for their delicious flavor and their numerous health promoting properties. Lychee are a rich source of vitamin C and B-complex which help to boost the immune system, protect against inflammation, and aid the body in metabolizing carbohydrates, proteins, and fats. Lychee contain a compound called oligonol which has powerful anti-viral properties and are highly beneficial for those suffering with colds, flu, fever, swollen glands, or sore throat. Lychees have the reputation of being able to help the most stubborn of coughs and provide significant respiratory relief from congestion and chronic coughs.

Lychee also contains flavonoids which can help to prevent the growth of cancer cells as well as reduce the size of tumors. Lychees are packed with antioxidants that are known to help reduce weight, improve circulation, and protect the body from aging and disease. Lychee also contains unique compounds that help to eliminate candida. Lychee is a good source of copper, iron, zinc, selenium, and potassium, which can help to nourish the blood and increase energy levels.

Lychee has a rough raspberry colored skin that can be easily peeled off to expose the juicy grape like fruit inside. Inside the juicy flesh is a shiny brown seed that should be discarded. The fruit is sweet and refreshing and is thoroughly enjoyed by children and adults alike. Fresh lychees are often found in the supermarket between July-October, but the fruit can also be found anytime of the year in the form of juices, jams, jellies, and sorbet. Dried or frozen lychee can also be found in specialty markets while healing lychee fruit extract can be found in capsule, tincture, tea, and liquid form online or at your local health food store.

Food Fact: Asparagus is high in glutathione, an important anti-carcinogen and is good source of vitamins A, C and E, B-complex vitamins, potassium and zinc. It also contains rutin, which protects small blood vessels from rupturing and may protect against radiation.

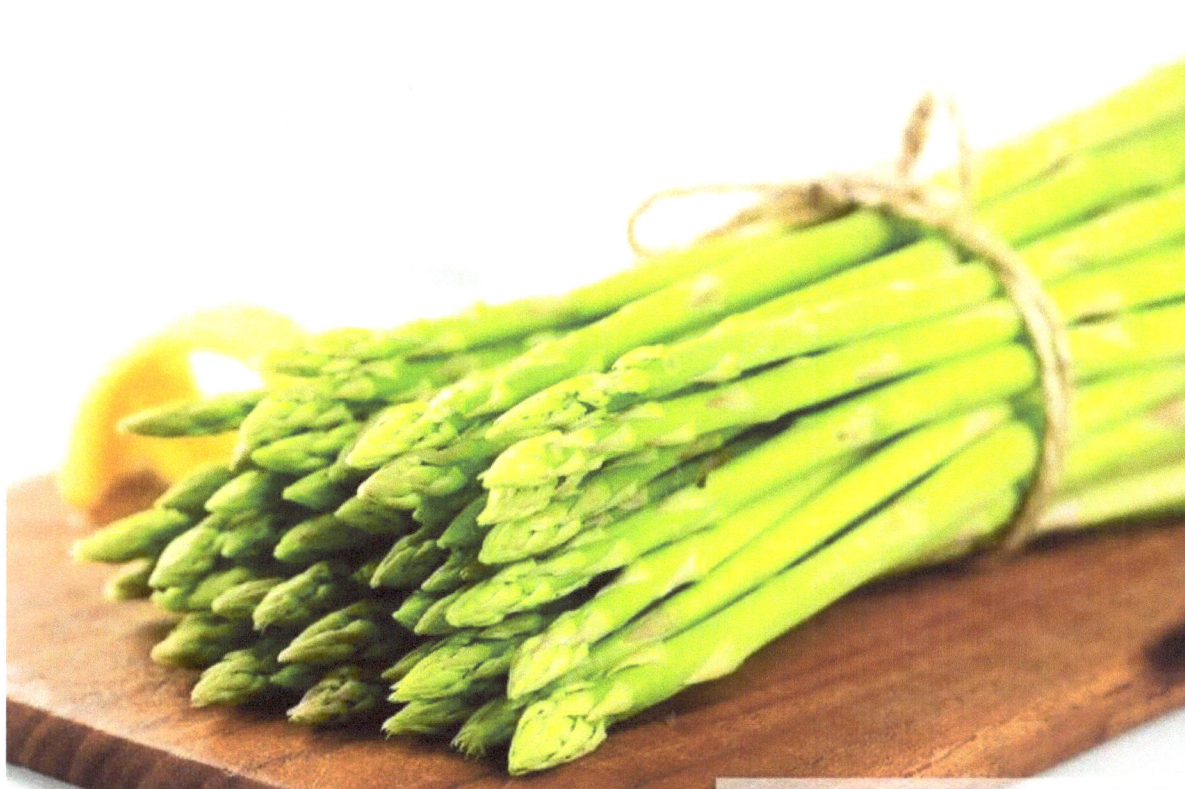

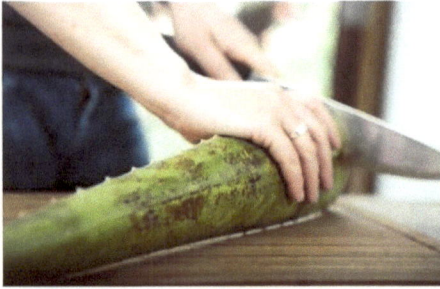

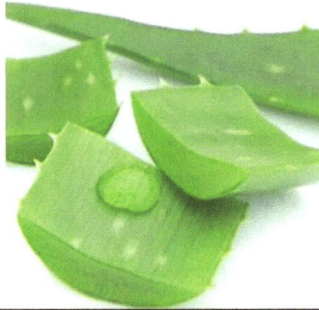

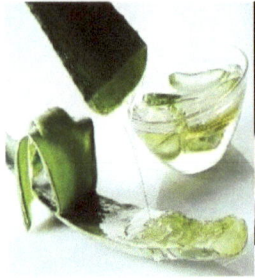

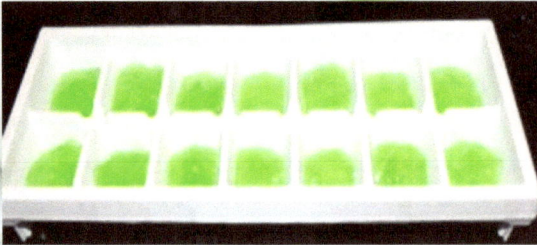

When I say aloe vera is the most impressive medicinal herb invented by nature, I don't make that statement lightly. Of all the herbs I've ever studied -- and I've written thousands of articles on nutrition and disease prevention -- aloe vera is the most impressive herb of them all. (Garlic would be a close second.) There is nothing on this planet that offers the amazing variety of healing benefits granted by aloe vera. In a single plant, aloe vera offers potent, natural medicine that:

• Halts the growth of cancer tumors.
• Lowers high cholesterol.
• Repairs "sludge blood" and reverses "sticky blood".
• Boosts the oxygenation of your blood.
• Eases inflammation and soothes arthritis pain.
• Protects the body from oxidative stress.
• Prevents kidney stones and protects the body from oxalates in coffee and tea.
• Alkalizes the body, helping to balance overly acidic dietary habits.
• Cures ulcers, IBS, Crohn's disease and other digestive disorders.
• Reduces high blood pressure natural, by treating the cause, not just the symptoms.
• Nourishes the body with minerals, vitamins, enzymes and glyconutrients.
• Accelerates healing from physical burns and radiation burns.
• Replaces dozens of first aid products, makes bandages and antibacterial sprays obsolete.
• Halts colon cancer, heals the intestines and lubricates the digestive tract.
• Ends constipation.
• Stabilizes blood sugar and reduces triglycerides in diabetics.
• Prevents and treats candida infections.
• Protects the kidneys from disease.
• Functions as nature's own "sports drink" for electrolyte balance, making common sports   drinks obsolete.
• Boosts cardiovascular performance and physical endurance.
• Speeds recovery from injury or physical exertion.
• Hydrates the skin, accelerates skin repair.

80

Anti Cancer Super fruits!
These are some of the fruits which might help you with cancer.

(Not complete treatment, but they can help you heal faster)

Anti-Cancer Superfruits

Nutrition Solution Lifestyle

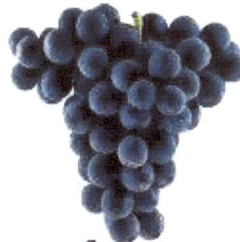
Grapes

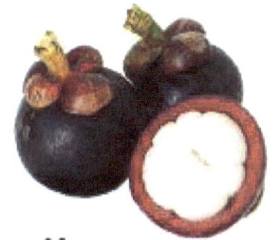
Mangosteen

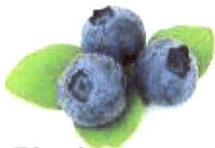
Blueberries

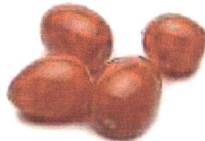
Goji Berries

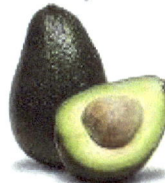
Avocado

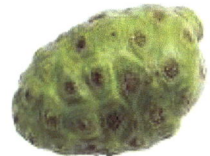
Noni

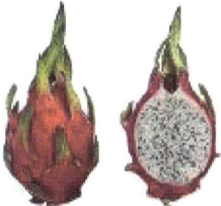
Dragon Fruit

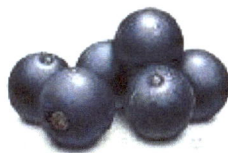
Acai Berries

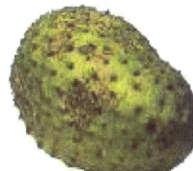
Soursop

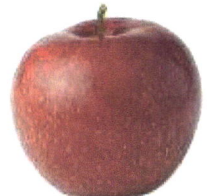
Apple

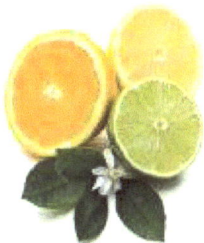
Citrus

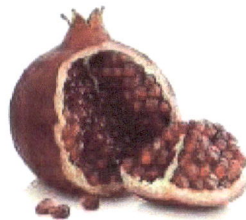
Pomegranate

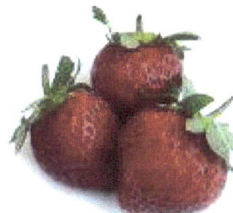
Strawberries

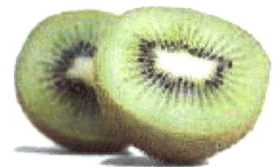
Kiwi

Is This Fruit Extract 10,000 Times Better Than Chemotherapy?

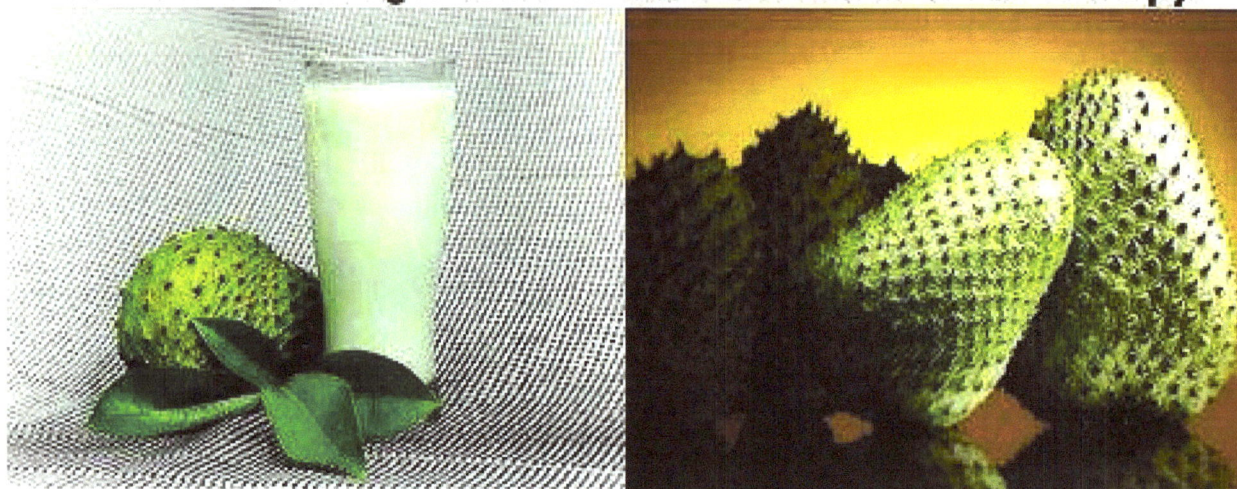

The Sour Sop or the fruit from the graviola tree is a miraculous natural cancer cell killer 10,000 times stronger than Chemo.

Please do share as much as you can, you can be the medium to save some one life (friends or family) or it could be your own.

Over a quarter of a century ago a study was performed on the seeds of the Soursop fruit, also known as graviola, which at that time demonstrated such amazing cancer-fighting potential, that those exposed to it within the conventional medical community looked upon it with complete incredulity.

Published in the Journal of Natural Products in 1996, Compound 1, one of five extracted from the seed of the graviola fruit, was found to be "selectively cytotoxic to colon adenocarcinoma cells (HT-29) in which it was 10,000 times the potency of adriamycin."

Adriamycin is the trade name for the chemoagent doxorubucin and is known by the nickname "red devil," due to both its deep red color and terrible side effects, which include life-threatening, even fatal damage to the cardiovascular system. This abject lack of "selective cytotoxicity," the ability to kill only the cancer cells and not healthy ones, is what makes Adriamycin so dangerous. And yet, it has been a first line treatment for a wide range of cancers for almost half a century.

Since the 1996 study, little research on graviola was performed. There was a cell study in 1999 which showed it had anti- prostate cancer and breast cancer activity; another 2002 cell study showed that graviola exhibited anti-hepatoma (liver cancer) activity, but nothing as promising as the original 1996 study ever followed.

Then, in 2011, the journal Nutrition and Cancer revealed highly promising research on Graviola and breast cancer. Researchers found that graviola fruit extract (GFE) suppressed so-called oncogene (or cancer-causing gene) expression in the cell and animal models of breast cancer. The oncogene known as epidermal growth factor receptor (EGFR) is commonly over-expressed in breast cancer, and therefore an ideal target for therapy.

According to the researchers

"A a 5-wk dietary treatment of GFE (200 mg/kg diet) significantly reduced the protein expression of EGFR, p-EGFR, and p-ERK in MDA-MB-468 [breast cancer] tumors by 56%, 54%, and 32.5%, respectively. Overall, dietary GFE inhibited tumor growth, as measured by wet weight, by 32% ($P < 0.01$)." [emphasis added]

The study authors concluded

"These data showed that dietary GFE induced significant growth inhibition of MDA-MB-468 cells in vitro and in vivo through a mechanism involving the EGFR/ERK signaling pathway, suggesting that GFE may have a protective effect for women against EGFR-overexpressing BC [breast cancer]." [emphasis added]

Given these findings the time may be ripe for reconsideration of graviola in the prevention and/or treatment of cancers, such as colon and breast cancer.

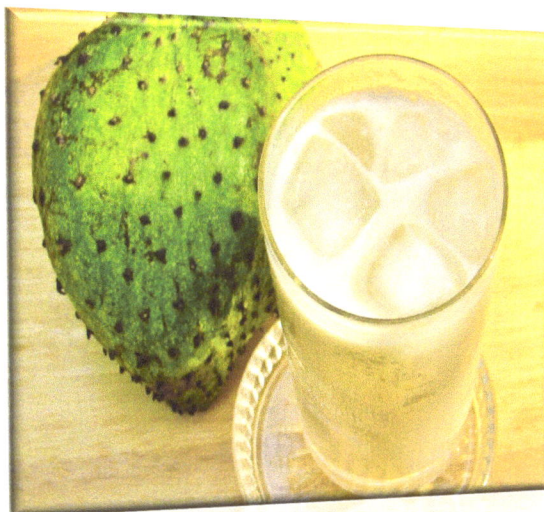

FOODS THAT CONTAIN CALCIUM

Broccoli	Bok Choy	Almonds	Pumpkin Seeds	Okra	Collards
Turnip Greens	Prickly Pear	Kohlrabi	Leeks	Brazil Nuts	Artichokes
Avocado	Celery	Green Beans	Coconut Meat	Onions	Gooseberry
Fennel	Dandelion Greens	Swiss Chard	Spinach	Kale	Butternut Squash
Brussels Sprouts	Mulberry	Cabbage	Sapote	Sesame Seeds	Asparagus

RawForBeauty

Celery is a strongly alkaline food that helps to counteract acidosis, purify the bloodstream, aid in digestion, prevent migraines, relax the nerves, reduce blood pressure, and clear up skin problems. Celery contains compounds called coumarins which are known to enhance the activity of certain white blood cells and support the vascular system. Celery's rich organic sodium content has the ability to dislodge calcium deposits from the joints and holds them in solution until they can be eliminated safely from the kidneys. Celery is a well known natural diuretic and has ample ability to flush toxins out of the body. Celery also has significant anti-inflammatory properties making it an essential food for those who suffer from auto-immune illnesses. It also contains significant amounts of calcium and silicon which can aid in the repair of damaged ligaments and bones. Celery is rich in vitamin A, magnesium, and iron which all help to nourish the blood and aid those suffering from rheumatism, high blood pressure, arthritis, and anemia. Fresh celery juice is one of the most powerful and healing juices one can drink. Just 16 oz of fresh celery juice a day can transform your health and digestion in as little as one week.

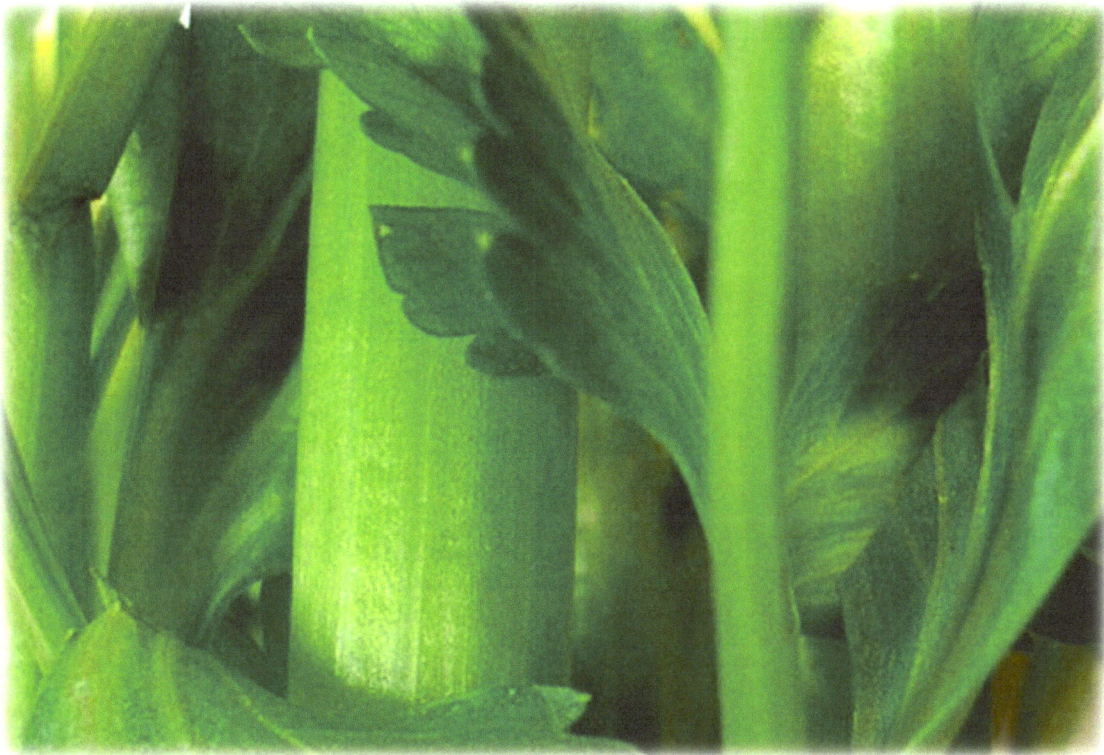

4 SUPERFOODS to incorporate into our lives for NUTRITION & NOURISHMENT

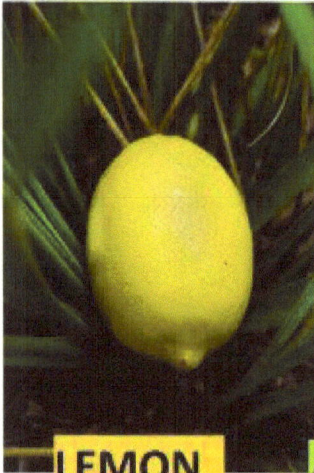

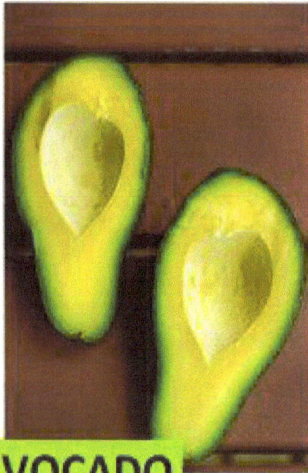

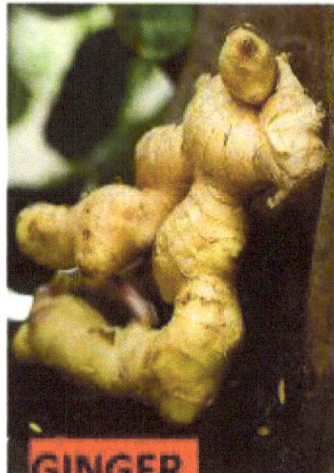

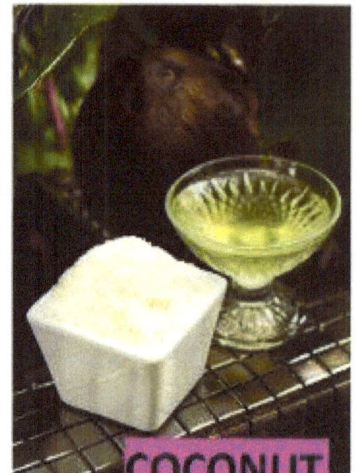

LEMON

1. Aids in Detoxing and Digestion

2. Burns fat and accelerates weight loss

3. High in Vitamin C

4. Relieves constipation

5. Alkalizes the body

AVOCADO

1. Good Healthy fats that aid in weight loss and burn fat!

2. Prevents & assists arthritis

3. Reduces and Reverses Aging

4. High in Vitamins A,C,K & B6

5. High in Fiber, Potassium & Folic Acid

GINGER

1. Rids Colds and Flus

2. Aids in weight loss and detoxification

3. High in Magnesium and Relieves muscle pain

4. Reduces inflammation

5. Relieves migraines & headaches

COCONUT

1. Accelerates Weight Loss

2. Lowers Cholesterol

3. Improves Diabetes

4. Aids digestion

5. A great natural skin Moisturizer

6. High in protein & calcium

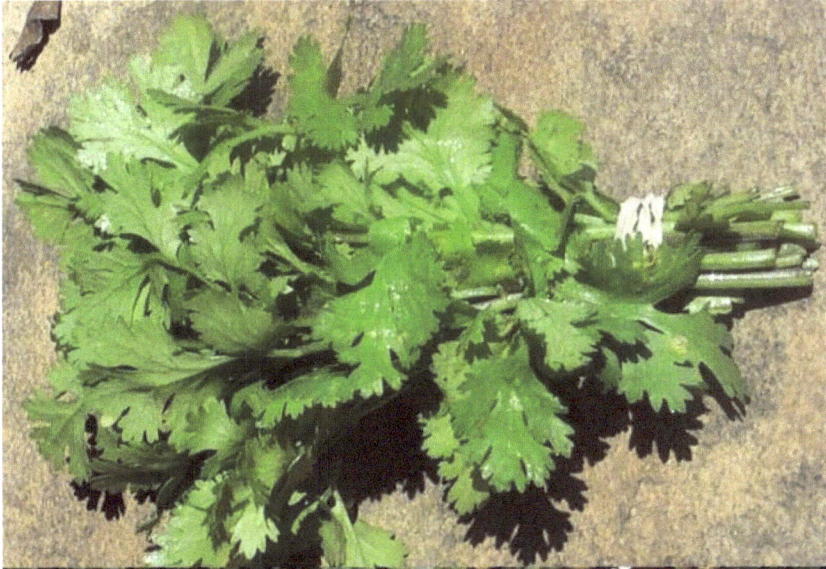

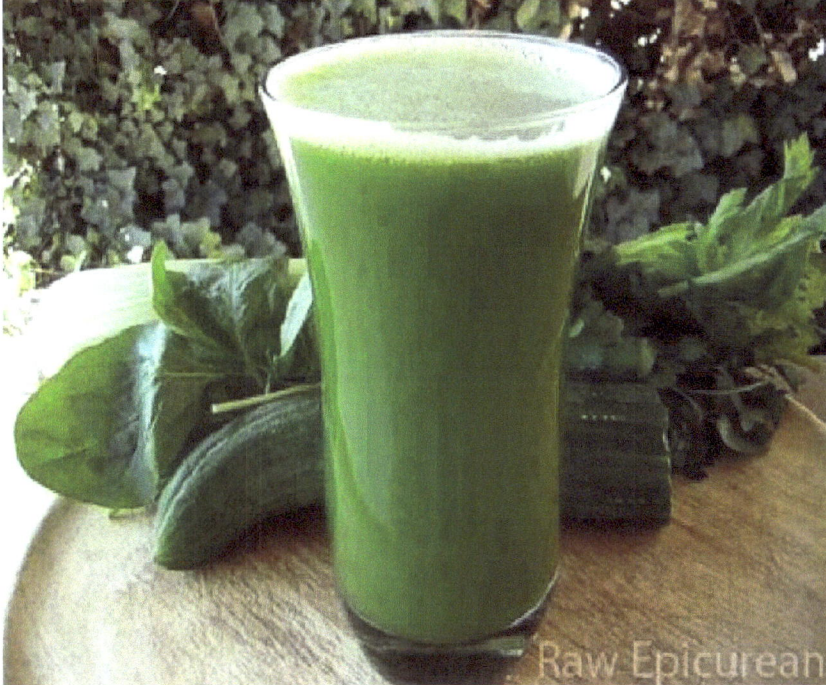

Years pass by and our kidneys are filtering the blood by removing salt, poison and any unwanted entering our body. With time, the salt accumulates and this needs to undergo cleaning treatments and how are we going to overcome this?

It is very easy, first take a bunch of parsley or Cilantro (Coriander Leaves) and wash it clean Then cut it in small pieces and put it in a pot and pour clean water and boil it for ten minutes and let it cool down and then filter it and pour in a clean bottle and keep it inside refrigerator to cool.

Drink one glass daily and you will notice all salt and other accumulated poison coming out of your kidney by urination also you will be able to notice the difference which you never felt before.

Parsley (Cilantro) is known as best cleaning treatment for kidneys and it is natural!

NOTE: We Are Only Providing You Information, Consult with your physician before taking supplements and adding herbs to your dietary intake.

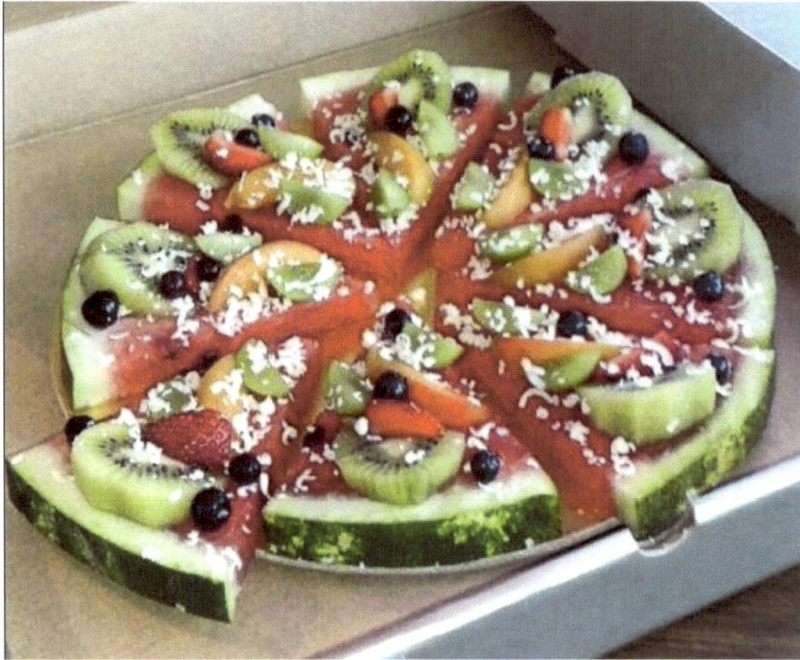

Kiwi fruit is exceptionally high in vitamin C, in fact it contains even more vitamin C than an orange. It also contains high amounts of vitamins E, A, & K as well as flavonoids, antioxidants, and minerals such as magnesium, potassium, and iron. Kiwi is particularly beneficial for the respiratory system and has been shown to help shorten the duration of colds as well as to help prevent asthma, wheezing, and coughing. Kiwi fruit contains anti-inflammatory properties which is good for those who suffer with autoimmune disorders such as Lupus, Fibromyalgia, CFS, and Lyme disease. Kiwi seeds are an excellent source of omega-3 fatty acids which are essential for cognitive function and can help prevent the development of ADHD and autism in children.

Kiwi contains enzymes similar to those in papaya and pineapple, which makes them useful in aiding in digestion and elimination. Kiwi fruit has also been shown to help protect DNA from mutating which is an incredible form of protection against illnesses and diseases such as atherosclerosis, heart disease, osteoarthritis, asthma, rheumatoid arthritis, and cancer. Kiwi fruit is also known to help remove excess sodium buildup in the body which can help reduce bloating, swelling, and water retention. Kiwi is good for promoting eye health and for preventing age-related macular degeneration.

It is also highly beneficial for those who have weak or sensitive immune systems and are useful at keeping ear, nose, and throat infections at bay. Kiwi is also great for diabetics by helping to keep their blood sugar levels under control and for cardiovascular health as it has been shown to help lower triglycerides or blood fat in the body.

Kiwi contains certain compounds that act as a blood thinner, similar to the way aspirin works which helps prevent blood clot formation inside the blood vessels and can protect the body from stroke and heart attacks. Green kiwi is the most commonly available variety found in supermarkets, however a delicious variety called Gold Kiwi (which has a golden color flesh) is a much sweeter, creamier, and less acidic variety that should not be missed. Kiwi fruit should be left on the counter to ripen until they yield under gentle pressure, like a ripe mango or avocado. Eat at least 3-4 ripe kiwi fruit a day for ultimate health benefits.

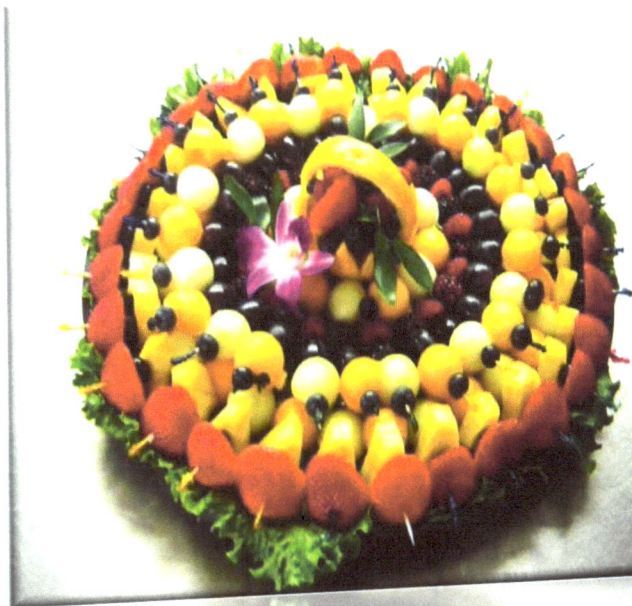

Spearmint is a sweet, mild herb that is packed with vitamins, minerals, and antioxidants such as vitamin A, C, B-complex, beta carotene, iron, magnesium, calcium, manganese, and potassium. Spearmint is wonderful for digestive ailments such as nausea, indigestion, ulcers, halitosis, and flatulence. It can also provide relief from headaches, sinus congestion, sore throats, fatigue, stress, and anxiety. Spearmint can also help to promote blood circulation and improve metabolism making it an excellent choice for cleansing and weight loss. Spearmint is also beneficial for respiratory issues such as bronchitis, asthma, and respiratory inflammation. If you are fortunate enough to have fresh spearmint on hand, try adding a few leaves to your smoothie or your fruit salad. It is a delicious flavor combination and provides an added mineral and antioxidant boost! Dried spearmint leaves are available online or in your local health food store and can be made into a refreshing herbal tea that can be taken either hot or cold on a daily basis for therapeutic benefits.

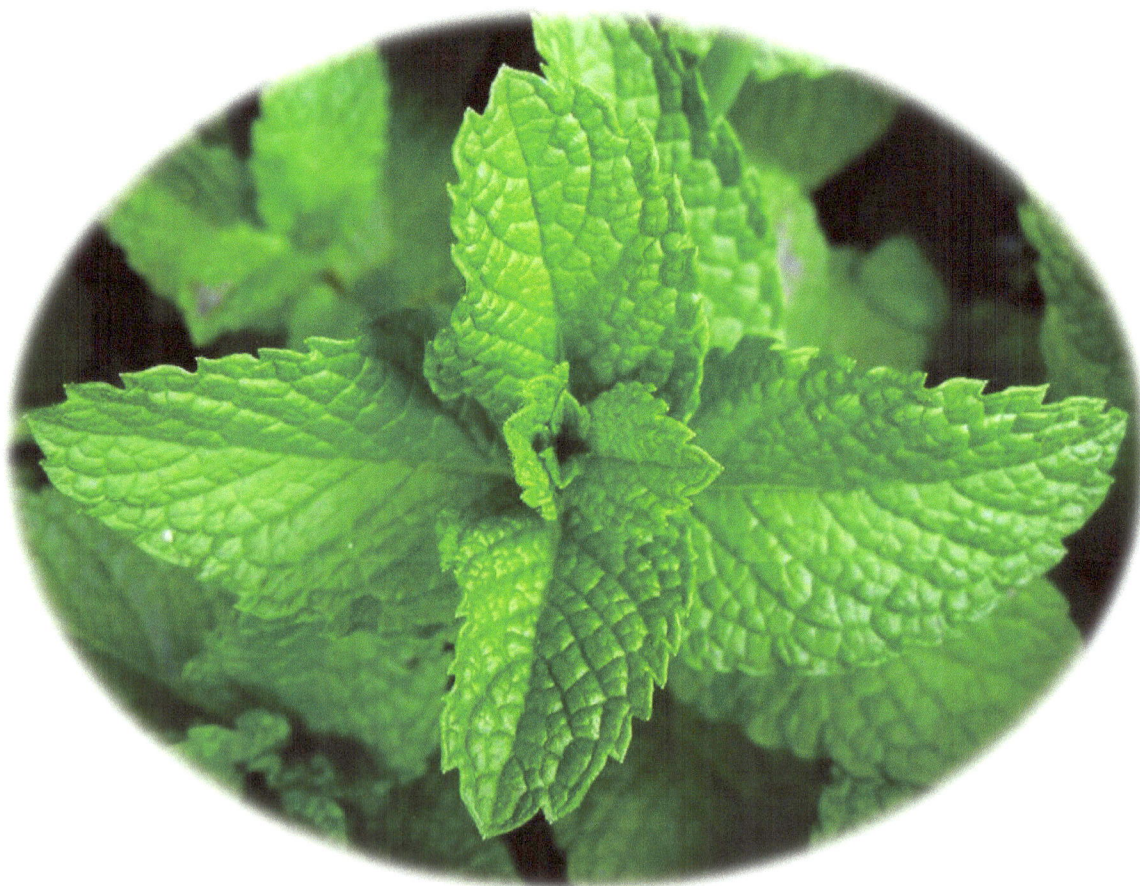

Fat Flush

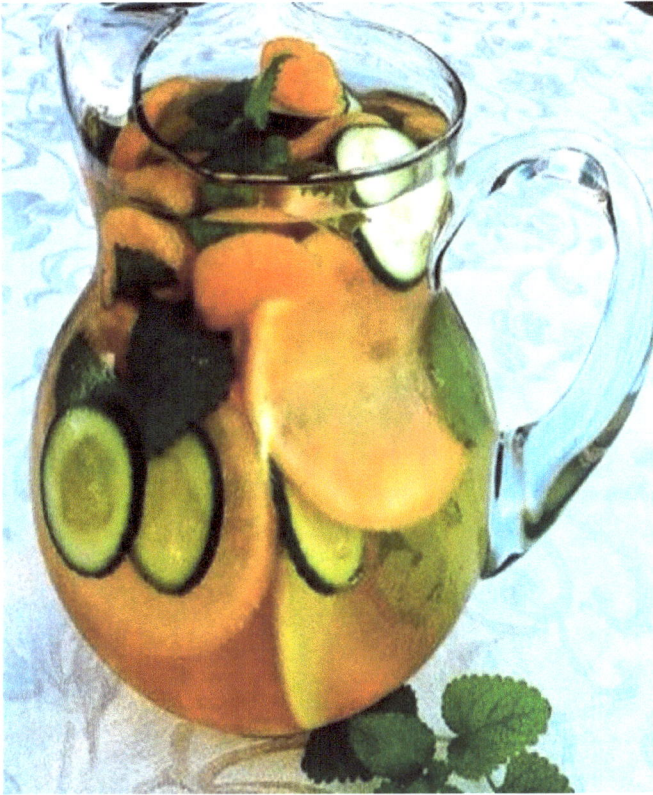

This is a very good fat flush and it is good for anyone that is taking skinny fiber to help flush fat and toxins out of your body....
If you can't have grapefruit, use lemon. If you can't find Tangerine, use an Orange.

REFRESHING FAT FLUSH WATER!!!...

You should drink at least half of your body weight in ounces per day, they say the longer it sits, the better it tastes. You can eat the fruit, etc., as well but they are intended as flavoring and still works, so that is a personal choice.

The Vitamin C turns fat into fuel, the tangerine increases your sensitivity to insulin, and the cucumber makes you feel full. Try it for 10 days and see what you think!

Ingredients per 8 oz serving

Water

1 grapefruit - or lemon

1 tangerine - or orange

½ cucumber, sliced

2 peppermint leaves

Ice – as much as you like

Directions
Wash the grapefruit, tangerine cucumber and peppermint leaves. Slice cucumber, grapefruit and tangerine (or peel). Combine all ingredients (fruits, vegetables, 8 oz. water, and ice) into a large pitcher.

ღ৸₡ღ Don't keep this recipe for yourself; share the love because sharing is sexy!! *ღ৸₡ღ*

Nature's Flu Shot

Juice from 6 fresh lemons
1 bulb garlic
2 tablespoons of honey
2 teaspoons of ginger powder
3 cups of pineapple juice
1/4 teaspoon cayenne pepper

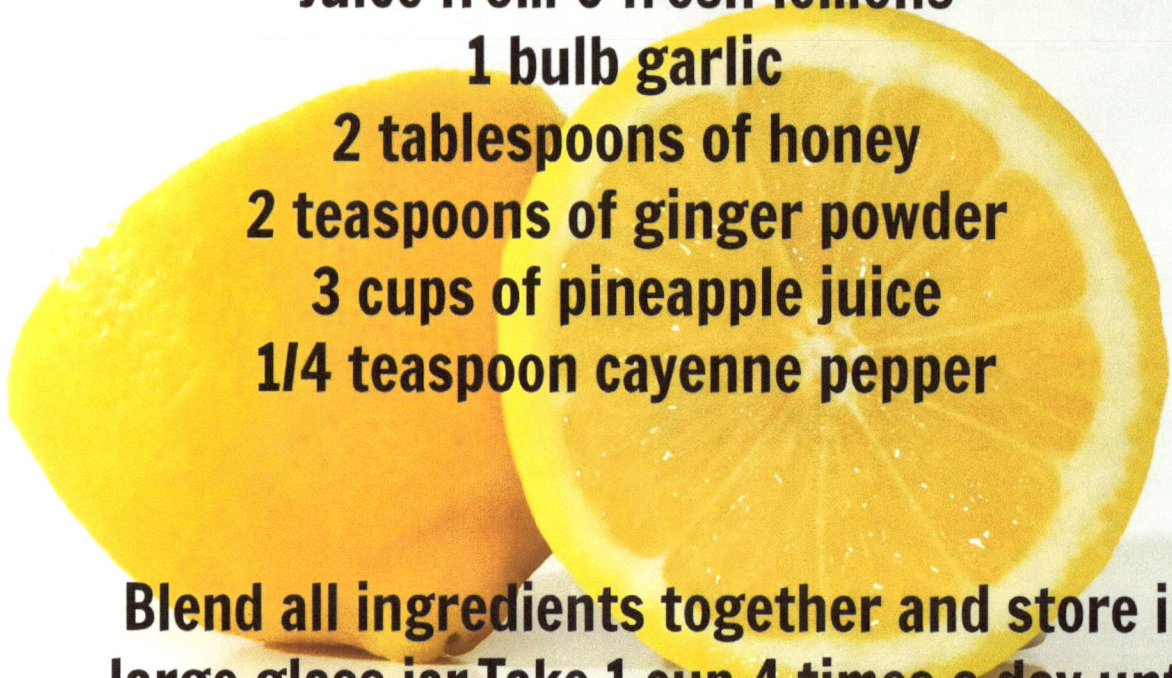

Blend all ingredients together and store in large glass jar.Take 1 cup 4 times a day until symptoms are gone.

Holistic, nutrient dense flu shot!

FLU SHOTS

~6 Kale Leaves~1/2 Bunch of Parsley ~1 Cucumber
~4 Celery Ribs~3 Small Apples~1/2 Lemon

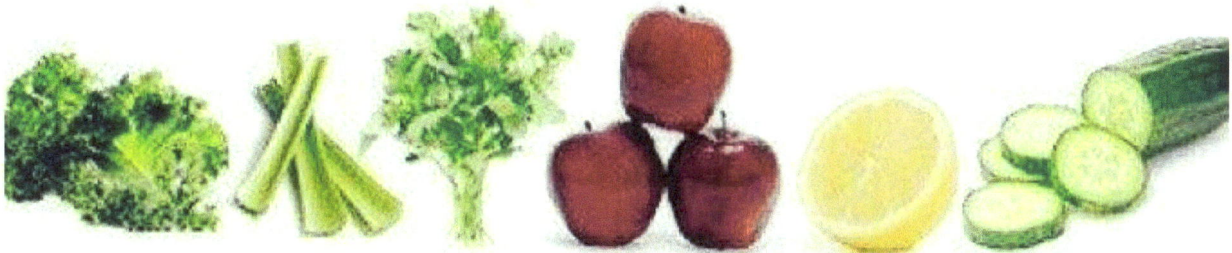

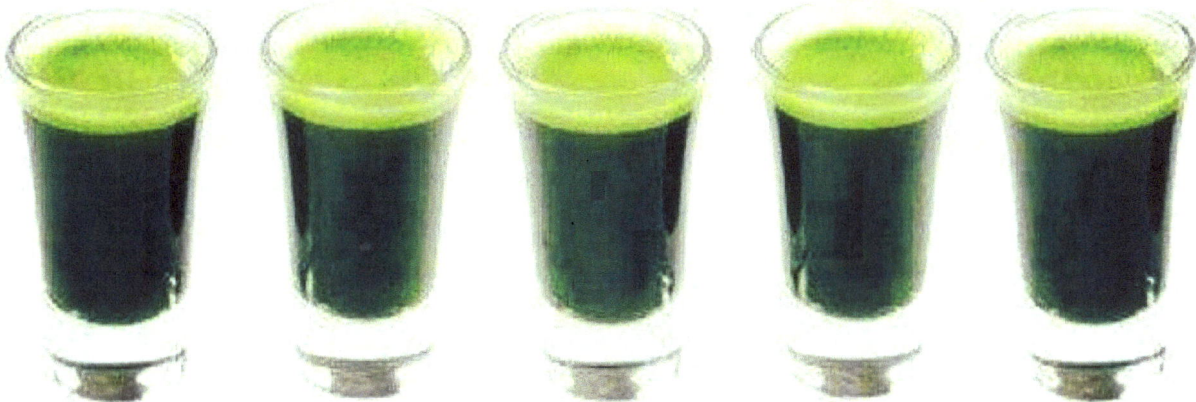

FOODS THAT HEAL THE KIDNEYS

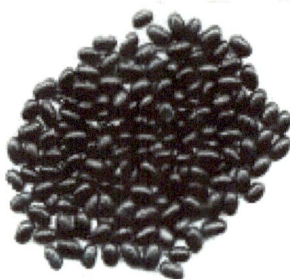

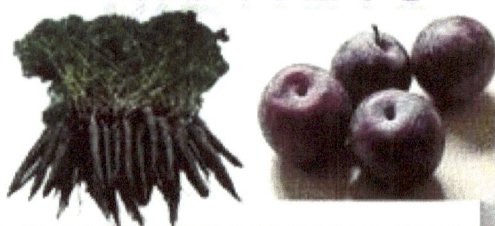

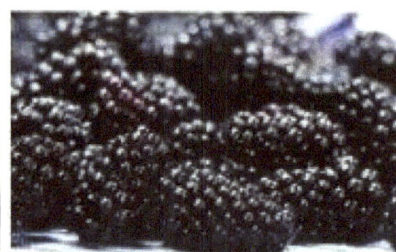

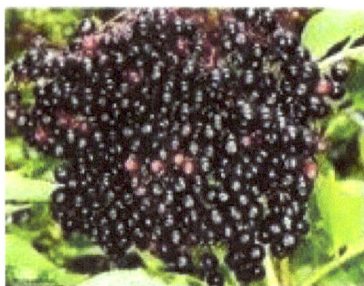

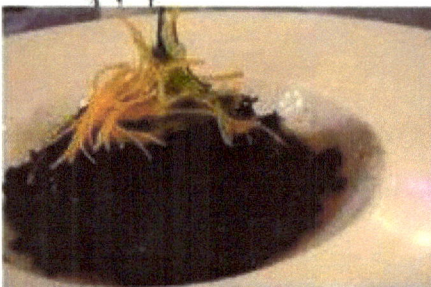

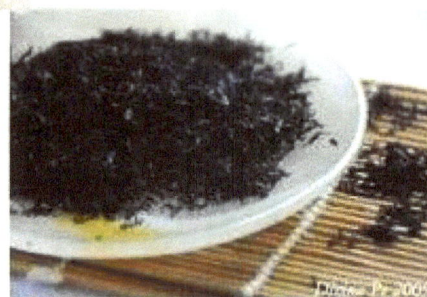

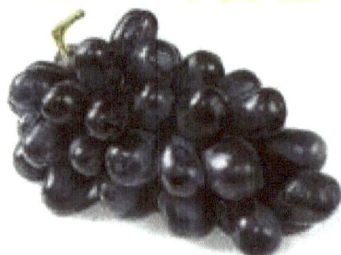

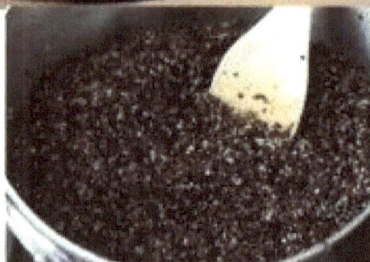

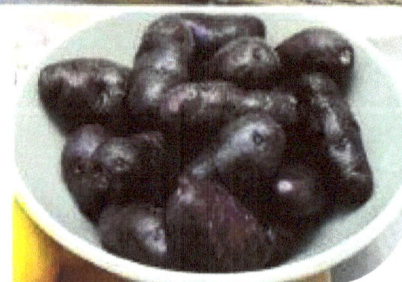

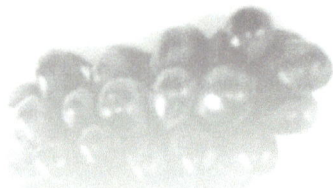

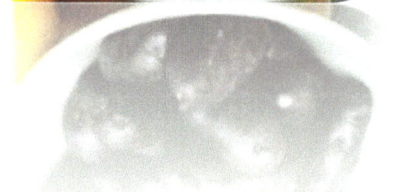

Black foods are the most POWERFUL in nutrients.

Powerful Health Info : Did You Know: Foods that heal the kidneys are purple plums, purple potatoes, black quinoa, blackberries, black carrots (purple carrots), hijiki (potent seaweed), black seaweed salad, black grapes, black beans, and black elderberries.

The blue, purple and indigo foods are great for their anti-aging properties. These foods have tons of antioxidants, which are called anthocyanins and phenolics. They help improve circulation and prevent blood clots, so they are great and can help prevent heart disease. They are also known to help memory function and urinary tract health and to reduce free radical damage.

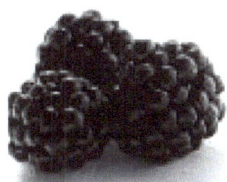
Blackberries

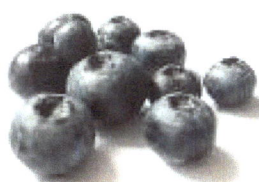
Blueberries

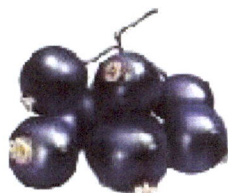
Black Currants

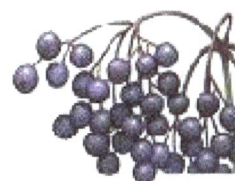
Elderberries

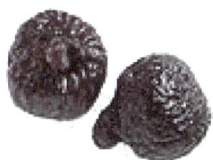
Figs

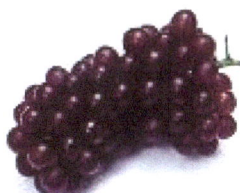
Purple Grapes

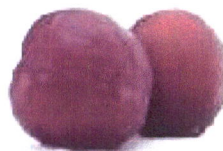
Plums

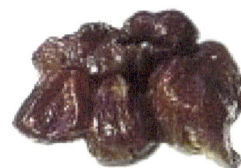
Prunes

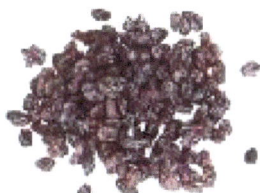
Raisins

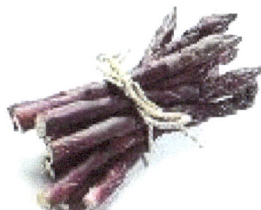
Purple Asparagus

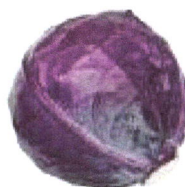
Purple Cabbage

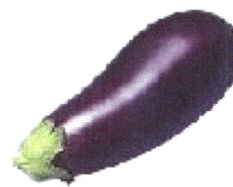
Eggplant

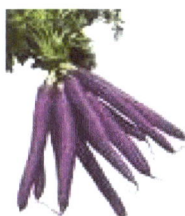
Purple Carrots

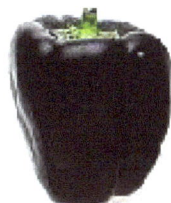
Purple Pepper

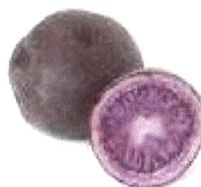
Purple Potatoes

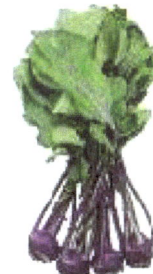
Purple Kohlrabi

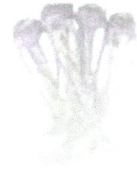

Make your own vitamin water. Add fruits instead of sugar for a natural sweetener for your H2O

Cut the fruit into paper-thin slices or small chunks. Combine ingredients with water. Refrigerate 4-6 hours. Serve over ice.

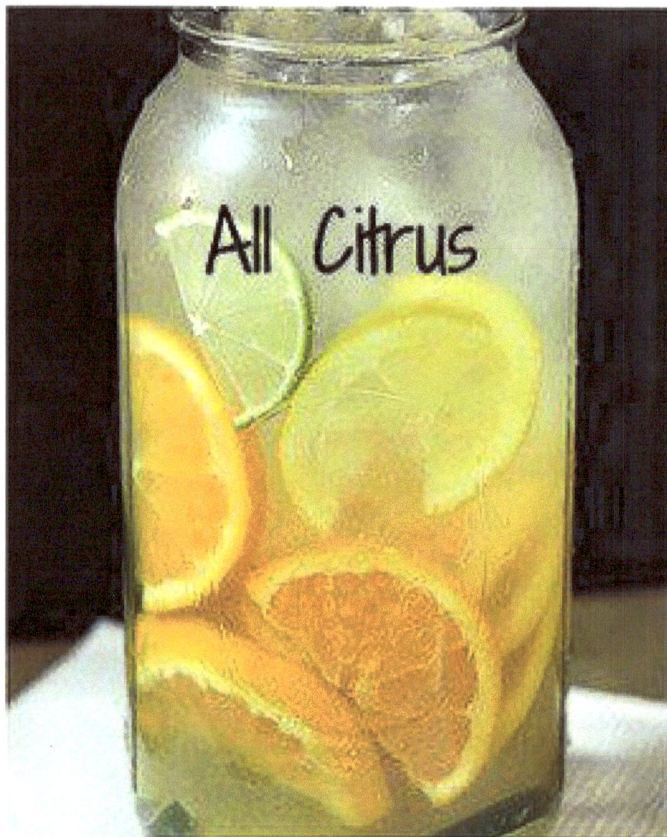

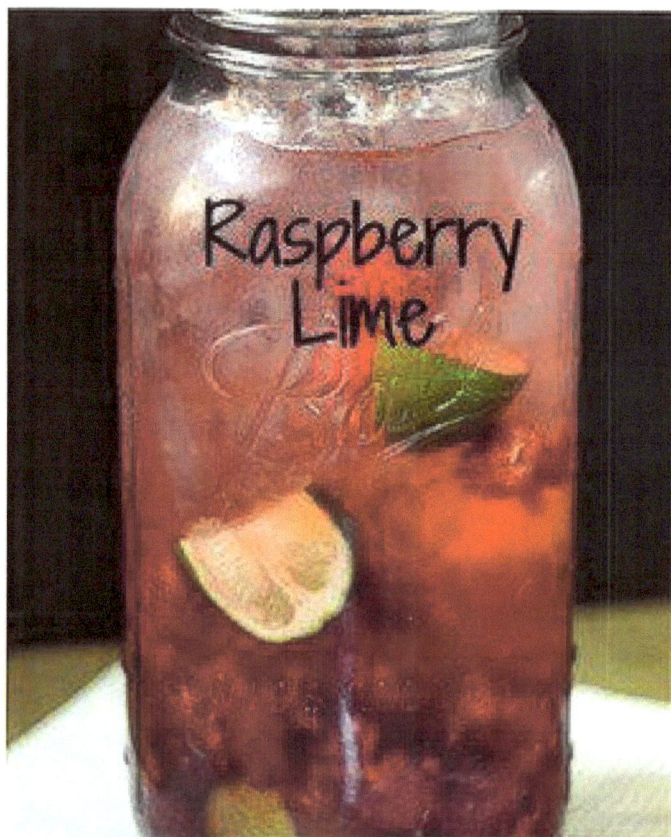

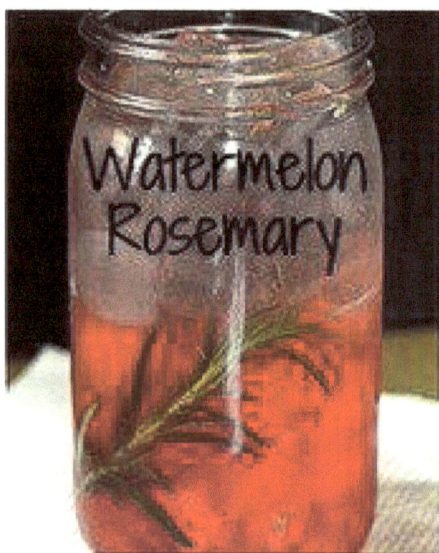

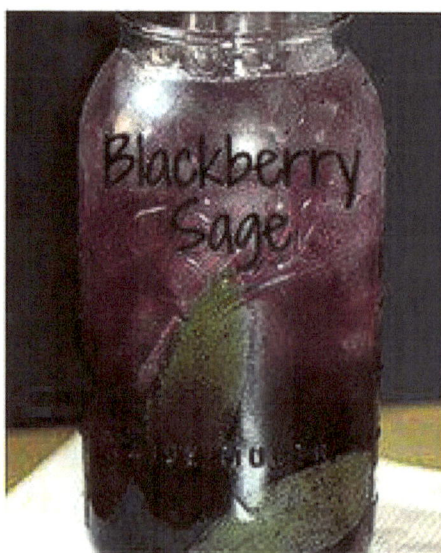

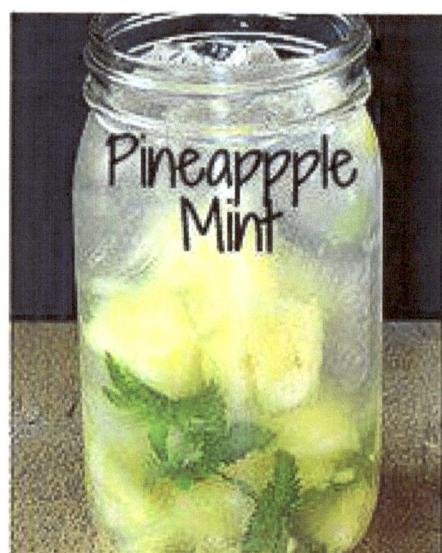

What is Hyaluronic Acid?

Hyaluronic acid (also called Hyaluronan) is a component of connective tissue whose function is to cushion and lubricate. Hyaluronan occurs throughout the body in abundant amounts in many of the places people with hereditary connective tissue disorders have problems such as joints, heart valves and eyes. Hyaluronic acid abnormalities are a common thread in connective tissue disorders. Interestingly, they are also common biochemical anomalies in most of the individual features of connective tissue disorders such as mitral valve prolapse, TMJ, osteoarthritis, and keratoconus.

Hyaluronic acid has been nicknamed by the press as the "key to the fountain of youth" because it has been noted that at least some people who ingest a lot of it in their diets tend to live to ripe old ages. ABC News had a show on a village in Japan and hyaluronic acid entitled, "The Village of Long Life: Could Hyaluronic Acid Be an Anti-Aging Remedy?". (It should be noted that the people in the ABC news show were thought to get high amounts of HA from starchy root vegetables their *natural diets*. They were not taking supplements.)

While a number of studies have linked abnormal levels of HA to either connective tissue disorders (CTDs) or conditions common in CTDs, such as premature aging, there are also a number of studies on Pubmed noting associations of high levels of HA to some forms of cancer. With HA as with other substances in the human body, such as estrogen and cholesterol, there are most likely optimal levels, and disease often occurs when these levels become out of range *in either direction*. Low estrogen levels have been linked to bone loss, while high estrogen levels have been associated with breast cancer. High cholesterol levels have been linked to heart attacks and stroke, while low levels have been linked to bleeding problems and depression. HA has been studied less than either cholesterol or estrogen, but the prudent path would be to assume that the body has optimal levels of HA, as it does for cholesterol, estrogen and many other substances.

As such, consult your doctor before you decide to take HA or any other type of supplement to make sure it is an appropriate treatment for your particular health condition.

Hyaluronic Acid and Connective Tissue Disorders

The list below contains links to a sample of the studies where subjects with connective tissue disorders have been shown to have hyaluronic acid (HA) abnormalities:

- Ehlers-Danlos syndrome
- Marfan syndrome
- Osteogenesis imperfecta
- Stickler syndrome

Not surprisingly, these disorders all have a lot of overlapping features, and many of these overlapping features, when studied individually, are also linked to hyaluronic acid abnormalities. In every study I looked at for connective tissue disorders that examined hyaluronic acid, the levels were always abnormal in patients with connective tissue disorders.

In human and animal studies, hyaluronic acid abnormalities occur in:

Heart valves with MVP
TMJ
Joint instability
Osteoarthritis
Detached retinas
Muscle contractures
Rachitic skeletal features (pectus excavatum, pectus carinatum, scoliosis, bowed limbs, hypermobility, etc.)
Glaucoma
Keratoconus
Poor scar formation (fetuses do not scar because of the high content of HA in amniotic fluid)
Acrogeria (prematurely wrinkled skin)
Fibromyalgia
Premature aging syndromes* (which share many features with connective tissue disorders, especially Ehlers-Danlos)

Hyaluronic acid, or commercial preparations containing hyaluronic acid, are in use, or being studied to be used, to prevent, treat or aid in the surgical repair for many the types of problems people with connective tissue disorders tend to have such as:

Fractures
Hernias
Glaucoma
Keratoconus
Detached retinas
Osteoarthritis (HA injections are the new breakthrough treatment for this condition)
Muscle contractures
TMJ
Prevents scarring
Vocal cord insufficiency
Wrinkled skin
Cartilage damage
Wound healing
Ligament Healing

The list below contains a partial list of common features of several connective tissue disorders. Both the syndromes and the individual features of the syndrome (even when the individual features are studied in the general population, not just in people with genetic disorders), all have links to hyaluronic acid abnormalities.

Syndrome with hyaluronic acid abnormalities	Features linked to *both* the syndrome and hyaluronic acid abnormalities
Ehlers-Danlos syndrome	mitral valve prolapse, prematurely wrinkled skin, pectus excavatum, pectus carinatum, scoliosis, bowed limbs, hypermobility, keratoconus, hernias, poor wound healing, joint instability, TMJ, contractures, osteoarthritis, fractures
Osteogenesis imperfecta	mitral valve prolapse, pectus excavatum, pectus carinatum, scoliosis, keratoconus, fractures, bowed limbs, hernias
Stickler syndrome	mitral valve prolapse, keratoconus, pectus excavatum, pectus carinatum, scoliosis, osteoarthritis, hypermobility, bowed limbs
Marfan syndrome	mitral valve prolapse, scoliosis, pectus excavatum, pectus carinatum, osteoarthritis, keratoconus, hypermobility, bowed limbs, hernias, detached retinas, glaucoma

Since the ABC special on hyaluronic acid called it the "Fountain of Youth", it is interesting that one of the defining characteristics of premature aging syndromes, such as Progeria, is hyaluronic acid abnormalities.

Related article:

Intra-articular Hyaluronic Acid Injections for Knee Osteoarthritis - Article from the American Academy of Family Physicians on beneficial effects of using HA for osteoarthritis.

Hyaluronic Acid and Environmental Factors

There are many factors known to influence hyaluronic acid levels. Genes are likely to be a factor, but there are many environmental factors that are known to have an impact, including zinc and magnesium availability. Not surprisingly, magnesium and zinc deficiencies are known to be associated with many of the same symptoms associated with hyaluronic acid abnormalities, such as mitral valve prolapse and poor wound healing, respectively. Perhaps this is because the zinc or magnesium deficiency contributes to the hyaluronic acid abnormality, which in turn causes the symptom.

There are a multitude of studies on Medline regarding hyaluronic acid and a wide variety of environmental factors. Here is a sample of some of the interesting ones that relate to connective tissue disorders:

Hyaluronic acid becomes abnormally elevated in the skin of swine who have zinc deficiencies. Magnesium is needed for hyaluronic acid synthesis. Perhaps a lack of magnesium is one of the factors in some connective tissue disorders. Magnesium supplementation is an established treatment for many of the symptoms of connective tissue disorders, such as fibromyalgia, mitral valve prolapse and contractures. (See my related topics on Magnesium and Mitral Valve Prolapse.)

Ascorbic acid can degrade hyaluronic acid. Estrogen treatment increases activity of hyaluronic acid. Estrogen is known to increase utilization of nutrients like magnesium and zinc - nutrients that are known to affect hyaluronic acid levels. Cigarette smoke is known to degrade hyaluronic acid.

In a study of rats, hyaluronic acid turnover and metabolism were affected by age, dietary composition, and caloric intake. If what rats ate affected their hyaluronic acid levels, then this may be a good clue that diet may well affect hyaluronic levels in humans, too. In another study on rats, hyaluronic acid deposition in rat cerebellum is affected by thyroid deficiency, thyroxine treatment and undernutrition. In a study of humans, hyaluronic acid levels were altered by physical activity and food ingestion.

In a study on rats, skin hyaluronic acid concentration was higher than normal in energy deficiency, but below normal levels in prolonged protein deficiency. In rats suffering from prolonged malnutrition, the collagen concentrations are reduced. (Reduced collagen concentrations are also found in some of the connective tissue disorders such as osteogenesis imperfecta, as are a plethora of other conditions also associated with hyaluronic acid abnormalities. Not surprisingly, zinc deficits are known to affect hyaluronic acid levels *and* are also known to cause reduced collagen levels in humans.)

Strep and staph bacteria emit an enzyme called hyaluronidase. Hyaluronidase is an enzyme which breaks down hyaluronic acid, thus allowing an entry point for the bacteria to enter the body. This may be why people may become hypermobile or develop heart aliments like mitral valve prolapse after illnesses such as rheumatic fever--because the hyaluronic acid in their connective tissue has been degraded by the bacteria that causes their illness. (See my section on "What Causes Mitral Valve Prolapse? Hyaluronic acid as a clue" for more on this topic.)

If animals that are genetically similar to humans such as rats can have reduced collagen levels and hyaluronic acid abnormalities from changes in their diets, then it would be logical to consider diet as a causative factor in people with the hyaluronic acid abnormalities.

Summary

Hyaluronic acid occurs in abundant amounts in many of the places people with connective tissue disorders have problems such as the joints, the eyes, the skin and heart valves. Hyaluronic acid is needed to cushion and lubricate joints, eyes, skin and heart valves.

People with connective tissue disorders and related features all seem to have abnormalities of hyaluronic acid. In every study I found that analyzed hyaluronic acid levels in people with connective tissue disorders or related disorders, when compared to controls they always had hyaluronic acid abnormalities.

HA is influenced by nutrition and other environmental factors. Many of the features of premature aging syndromes and connective tissue disorders are also known to be caused by nutritional deficiencies, and not surprisingly these are often the same nutritional factors that influence the manufacture of hyaluronic acid. My theory is that this is not all one big coincidence. Logically, it is more likely to be a predictable sequence of causes and effects.

Hyaluronic acid is being used commercially or experimentally to correct a large portion of the problems found in connective tissue disorders such as fractures, eye disorders, poor wound healing and prematurely wrinkled skin. It would be highly logical to consider the possibility that hyaluronic acid works to correct these problems because defects or deficiencies of hyaluronic acid are what cause these problems in the first place.

Perhaps controlling or optimizing the environmental factors, such as modifying ones diet, to optimize hyaluronic acid levels would be helpful in treating many inherited connective tissue disorders and premature aging syndrome.

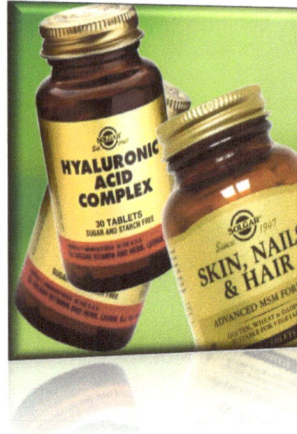

Key Benefits of Hyaluronic Acid Supplementation

- Hyaluronic acid (HA) moisturizes skin from the inside out, smoothing out wrinkles in the process. HA acts as an internal cosmetic to hydrate the skin.
- Hyaluronic acid is for people who need to ease the flexing of their joints, especially their knees, by restoring cushioning to their joints.
- Hyaluronic acid is for men and women in their 30s and 40s who are beginning to see the first signs of aging.
- Hyaluronic acid is for seniors who have established joint conditions.
- Studies show oral hylaronic acid supplementation provides these benefits to most people after administration for only 2 to 4 months.

Basic Functions of Hyaluronic Acid

As Hyaluronic Acid is present in every tissue of the body; hyaluronic acid's importance cannot be underestimated. Retention of water is one of the most important biological functions of hyaluronic acid, [1] second only to providing nutrients and removing waste from cells that do not have a direct blood supply, such as cartilage cells. With a lower than adequate amount of hyaluronic acid, nutrients cannot be moved into these cells and waste cannot be eliminated from cells. Hyaluronic acid is sometimes abbreviated as HA.

Hyaluronic acid is found in the synovial joint fluid, the vitreous humor of the eye, the cartilage, blood vessels, extracellular matrix, skin and the umbilical cord.

Hyaluronic Acid is Found in Synovial Joint Fluid

Our joints (like the elbows and knees) are surrounded by a membrane called the synovial membrane, which forms a capsule around the ends of the bones. This membrane secretes a liquid called the synovial fluid. Basically, the synovial fluid is found in joint cavities. It has many functions, including serving as a lubricant, shock absorber and a nutrient carrier. The fluid protects the joints and bones. Cartilage is immersed in the synovial fluid and is a fibrous connective tissue. Cartilage is avascular, meaning it contains no blood vessels. This is why the synovial fluid is so important. Synovial fluid is the only way in which nutrients can be carried into the cartilage and waste can be removed.

Hyaluronic Acid is a Key Component of Cartilage

Cartilage is a specialized form of connective tissue. Hyaline cartilage is the most predominant form of cartilage in the body. It lends strength and flexibility to the body. A key component of cartilage is hyaluronic acid. Cartilage is also avascular – with no blood vessels. Nutrients are brought by the synovial fluid, which is rich in hyaluronic acid to the cartilage, which is also hyaluronicacid rich.

Hyaluronic Acid is in the Extracellular Matrix

Hyaluronic Acid is found in the extracellular matrix (ECM). The ECM is composed of material (fibrous elements, including glycosamino-glycans) produced by the cells and excreted to the extracellular space with the tissues. All nutrients and metabolic waste are transported through the ECM. Hyaluronic acid is a major constituent of the ECM and serves as an essential structural element of the ECM. Hyaluronic acid locks moisture into the ECM and hyaluronic acid supports the structural integrity of the extracellular matrix.

Hyaluronic Acid in the Skin

In the skin, the extracellular matrix is composed of hyaluronic acid and other sulfated GAGs, combined with collagen and elastin. Large amounts of water are held in the ECM. When elastin is not bathed in water, it becomes dry and brittle, thus the look of dry, brittle, wrinkled skin.[1]

Half-life is defined as the time required for one half of the total amount of a particular substance to be consumed, broken down, or depleted. The half-life of hyaluronic acid in the cartilage is 2-3 weeks. But the half-life of hyaluronic acid in the skin is less than 1 day! Hyaluronic acid is present in both the dermis and the epidermis. 50% of the body's naturally produced hyaluronic acid that is found in the epidermis is metabolized and excreted in less than 24 hours. Like hyaluronic acid produced in the body, hyleronic acid taken as a nutritional supplement moisturizes from the dermis to the epidermis - from deeper layers of the skin to the outer layer.

The extracellular matrix fills up the space between the skin cells. This makes the skin soft, smooth and elastic. But as we age, hyaluronic content in the skin changes due to two separate clinically proven factors.

1. There is a decrease in synthesis of hyaluronic acid.

2. Recompartmentalization – from the epidermis to the dermis.

Both changes leave the epidermis depleted in hyaluronic acid resulting in thinning, aging, and decreased moisture in the skin.

Medical Treatment with Hyaluronic Acid

Hyaluronic acid for use by humans has been derived from rooster combs. Rooster combs provide the purest form of hyaluronic acid available.

Osteoarthritis Treatment
Physicians have injected hyaluronic acid directly into the synovial fluid in the knee as a treatment for osteoarthritis of the knee for the past 20 years. There are many peer-reviewed articles written on the use of hyaluronic acid extracted from rooster combs for this purpose. Cost is a concern. The wholesale cost for the hyaluronic acid treatment series is about $620, plus the cost of the outpatient facility and the physician.

From the Leaflet "Treating Knee Osteoarthritis with Injections" published by the American Academy of Family Physicians:

> "Your doctor might inject an anesthetic agent. This is a medicine that makes your knee numb. It can stop the pain for a short time--maybe days or a few weeks. Another medicine, called a corticosteroid, can be injected along with the anesthetic. These medicines together might make your pain stay away longer.

> "In the past few years, a medicine called hyaluronic acid has been used for knee injections. Some hyaluronic acid is already in the fluid in your joints. In people with osteoarthritis, the hyaluronic acid gets thinner. When this happens, there isn't enough hyaluronic acid to protect the joint like it used to. Injections can put more hyaluronic acid into your knee joint to help protect it."

Skin Treatment

Hyaluronic acid injection can be used to improve the skin's contour and reduce depressions in the skin due to acne, scars, injury or lines. Immediately or within a few hours after injection the site may be red and swollen. This usually disappears within a week. Another one or two treatments (at least a week apart) may be necessary to achieve the desired correction. Hyaluronic acid implantation is not permanent. Like natural hyaluronic acid, manufactured hyaluronic acid once injected into the skin will gradually break down and be absorbed by the body. In most cases, the hyaluronic acid augmentation usually lasts between 6-9 months. Compared to collagen implants hyaluronic acid appears to have a longer augmentation effect, possibly lasting 2 to 3 times longer than the average collagen implant. To maintain the initial results, repeat hyluronic acid injections or top-up treatments will be necessary. Most people following this protocol have 2 to 3 treatments per year.

Alternative Treatments

Alternative treatments which impact the hyaluronic acid in the skin include Retinoids prescribed by physicians which increase the natural synthesis of hyaluronic acid and accelerate the shedding of the skin. Chemical peels remove the top, dry layer(s) of the skin. Facials cleanse the pores and superficially moisturize the skin.

Nutritional Supplementation with Hyaluronic Acid

Hyaluronic acid extracted from rooster combs has too large a chemical size for absorption by the intestinal tract. When directly extracted from rooster combs, the molecular weight is 1.2 to 1.5 million Daltons (Da). For comparison, the average molecule weight of an amino acid is approximately 110 Da. But, wouldn't you know it, Japanese scientists developed a proprietary enzyme-cleaving technique to lower the molecular weight of hyaluronic acid without altering its chemical nature. The final molecular weight of hyaluronic acid processed by the Injuv™ process is 5,000 Daltons. This allows hyaluronic acid to be taken orally as a nutritional supplement.

Oral Hylauronic acid studies show benefits for most study participants when taken for a period of only 2 to 4 months. Patient reports indicate that continued use of hyaluronic acid sustain the benefits. Some patients are able to decrease the dose after the desired results are achieved.

Conclusion

- Hyaluronic acid is essential for the health of the synovial fluid which supports the bones and joints.
- Hyaluronic acid is essential for the structure of the extracellular matrix in the skin and to insure that the matrix has the ability to hold onto its essential fluid – hydration of the skin.
- The extracellular matrix in the skin keeps the skin moist and supple.
- The skin responds best with hyaluronic acid introduced from the inside out – from the dermis to the epidermis.
- Hyaluronic acid for supplementation is extracted from rooster combs. It is the purest form available.
- Proprietary processing by a method such as the Injuv™ method is done to produce low molecular weight hyaluronic acid which is absorbable through the intestinal tract.
- Supplementation with hyaluronic acid is crucial due to decreased synthesis or re-compartmentalization of hyaluronic acid that occurs with aging.

References

1. Block, A., and Bettelheim, F.: Water Vapor Sorption of Hyaluronic Acid, Biochim Biophys Acta 201, 69, 1970
2. Goa K. L. and Benfield P.: Drugs 1994, 47: 536-566.
3. Laurent, T., and Gergely, J.: Light Scattering Studies on Hyaluronic Acid, J Biol Chem 212, 325, 1955.
4. George E. Intra-articular hyaluronan treatment for osteoarthritis. Ann Rheum Dis 1998;57:637-40.
5. Wobig M, Bach G, Beks P, Dickhut A, Runzheimer J, Schwieger G, et al. The role of elastoviscosity in the efficacy of viscosupplementation for osteoarthritis of the knee: a comparison of hylan G-F 20 and a lower-molecular-weight hyaluronan. Clin Ther 1999;21:1549-62.
6. Weiss C, Balazs EA, St. Onge R, Denlinger JL. Clinical studies of the intraarticular injection of HealonR (sodium hyaluronate) in the treatment of osteoarthritis of human knees. Osteoarthritis symposium. Palm Aire, Fla., October 20-22, 1980. Semin Arthritis Rheum. 1981;11(suppl 1):143-4.
7. New Zealand Dermatological Society, Dec 2, 2002.

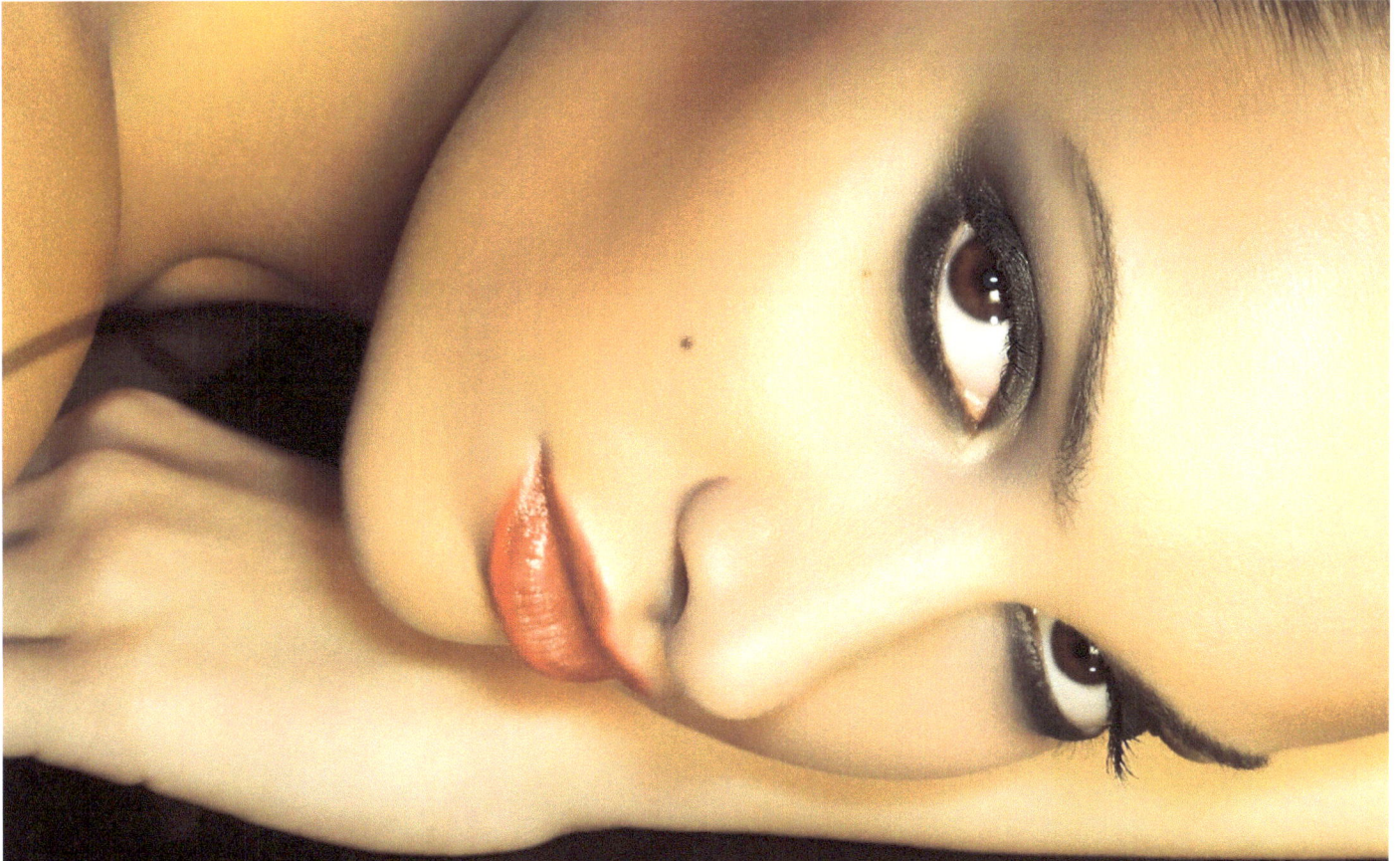

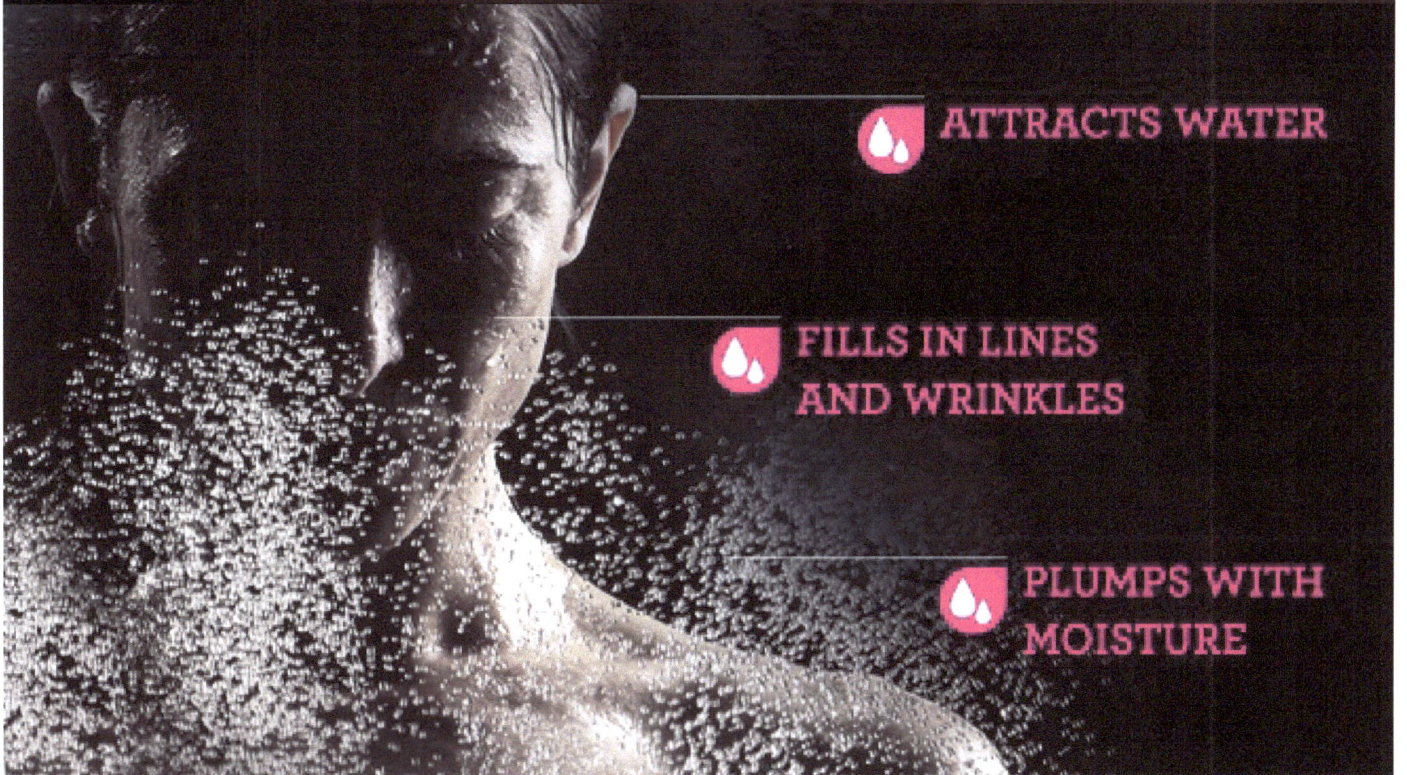

ATTRACTS WATER

FILLS IN LINES
AND WRINKLES

PLUMPS WITH
MOISTURE

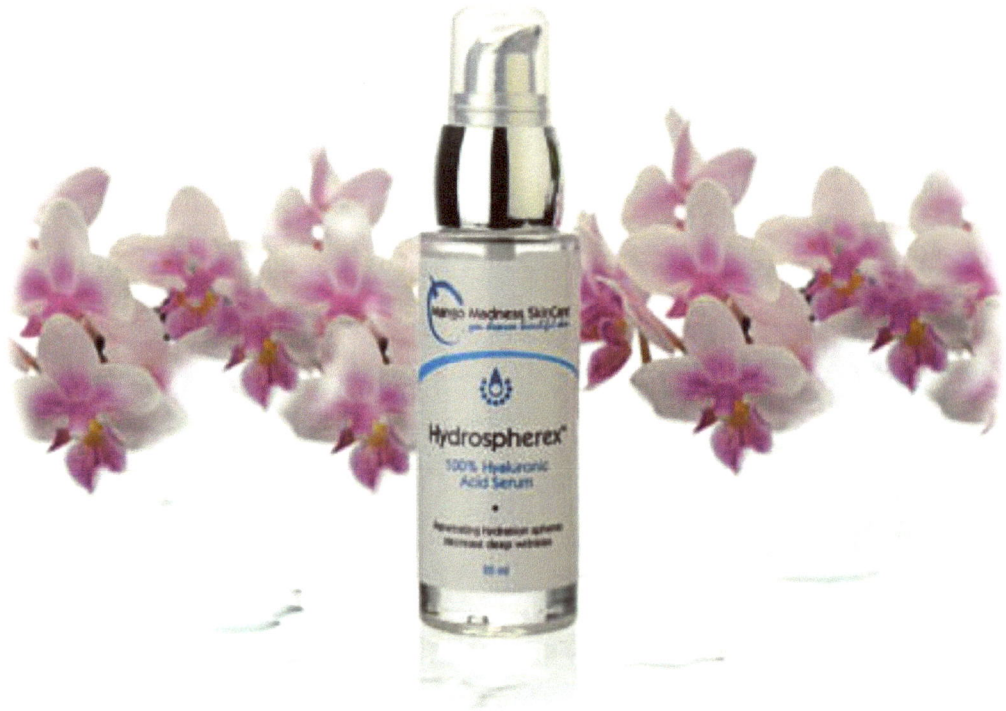

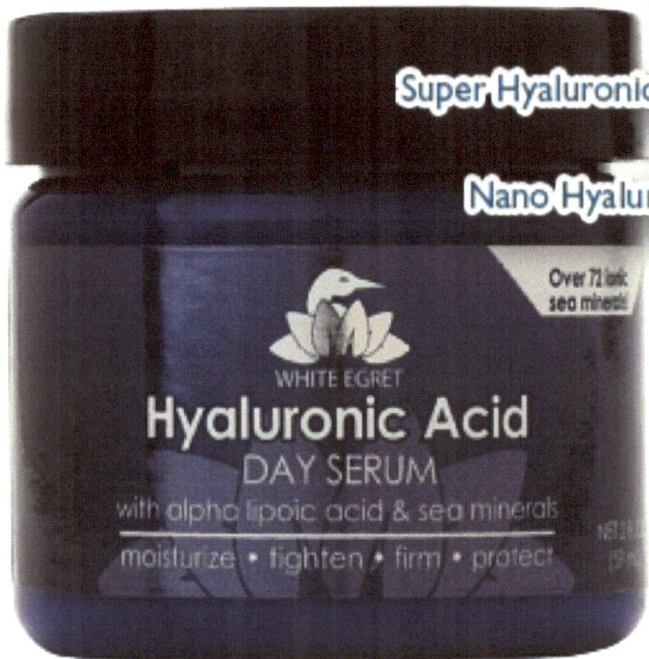

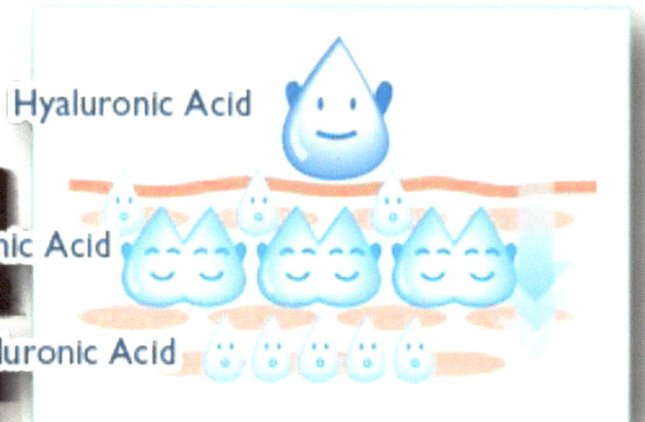

Hyaluronic Acid

Super Hyaluronic Acid

Nano Hyaluronic Acid

108

Notes

Notes

Notes

Notes

Notes

Notes

Notes

Notes

Notes

Notes

Notes

Notes

Notes

Notes

Notes

Notes

Notes

Notes

Notes

Notes